# SOMATIC EXERCISES FOR WEIGHT LOSS

Ultimate Guide to Low Impact Exercises to Increase Flexibility, Relief Stress and Emotional Well-being

**CHARLES K BENAVIDES**

# TABLE OF CONTENT


**INTRODUCTION**...............................................................**8**

Understanding Somatic Exercises......................... 11

Somatic Movement's Benefits for Losing Weight... 12

**CHAPTER 1**.............................................................. **16**

**THE RELATIONSHIP BETWEEN THE MIND AND BODY**................................................................... **16**

Examining the Relationship Between Mind and Body in Weight Loss................................................. 17

How Somatic Exercises  Impact Body Awareness. 19

**CHAPTER 2**.............................................................. **23**

**FUNDAMENTALS OF SOMATIC TRAINING**............. **23**

Fundamental Ideas in Somatic Movement............. 24

Methods for Including Somatic Exercises in Everyday Activities...............................................26

**CHAPTER 3**.............................................................. **30**

**WEIGHT LOSS AND BREATHWORK**.........................**30**

Breath: An Essential Part of Somatic Practices......31

Breathing Techniques for Relaxation and Stress Reduction............................................................33

**CHAPTER 4**.............................................................. **38**

**SOMATIC ACTIVITIES TO INCREASE FLEXIBILITY AND MOBILITY**.......................................................**38**

Mild Motions to Enhance Joint Flexibility............... 39

Stretching Patterns to Increase Flexibility............44

**CHAPTER 5**.............................................................. **52**

**RELEASING STRESS AND TENSION**...................... **52**

Physical Methods to Reduce Stress......................53

Using Somatic Practices to Address Emotional

Eating.................................................................57

**CHAPTER 6**..................................................... **62**

**SOMATIC EXERCISES FOR STRENGTHENING THE CORE**.................................................. **62**

Abdominal Toning and Sculpting Exercises............67

**CHAPTER 7**..................................................... **74**

**ADJUSTING POSTURE TO LOSE WEIGHT**.............. **74**

The Impact of Posture on Weight Management..... 75

Physical Activities to Enhance Postural Alignment.78

**CHAPTER 8**..................................................... **83**

**SOMATIC AWARENESS AND MINDFUL EATING**..... **83**

Developing Insightfulness in Eating Behaviors.......84

Improving Eating Awareness Through Somatic Practices............................................................87

**CHAPTER 9**..................................................... **91**

**INCLUDING SOMATIC EXERCISES IN YOUR DAILY ROUTINE**........................................................ **91**

Guides for Success and Maintenance Over the Long Term...................................................................95

**CONCLUSION**.................................................. **99**

Key Concepts Recap:.........................................99

Encouragement for Continued Somatic Practice for Weight Loss..................................................... 102

**A 14-DAY WORKOUT PLAN**...............................**107**

14-Day Somatic Exercise Plan for Weight Loss... 107

## Scan QR Code to Access Free Bonuses and Join Our 30 Day Challenge.

## HOW TO SCAN QR CODE

To scan a QR code, take the following general actions:

**1. Open the Camera App**: The majority of contemporary smartphones come with a built-in QR code scanning feature in their camera apps. Open the camera app on your smartphone.

**2. Set the Camera Position**: Slightly shake your phone and aim the camera toward the QR code you wish to scan. Verify that the well-lit QR code is inside the frame.

**3. Scan the QR Code**: The QR code ought to be instantly recognized by your smartphone's camera app. It could provide a link or a notification to access the content linked to the QR code.

4. **Follow the Prompt**: After the QR code is detected, adhere to any on-screen instructions. This could include clicking on a link to visit a website, downloading an application, or seeing particular content.

**5. Access the Content**: You ought to be able to view the content linked to the QR code after scanning it and following any instructions. This might be a website, an electronic voucher, contact details, or other kinds of information.

You might need to enable the QR code recognition option in your smartphone's settings or download a QR code scanning app from the app store if the camera app on your phone isn't picking up codes automatically. You should consult your device's user manual for more details since certain devices might have unique motions or instructions for reading QR codes.

# INTRODUCTION

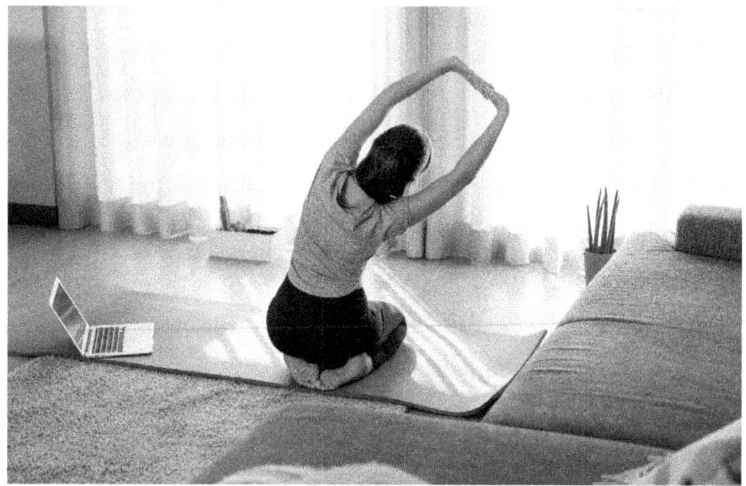

In a society where quick cures, fad diets, and intense workout regimens all promise instant weight loss, the real meaning of health and well-being is sometimes lost in the shuffle. Somatic activities are a gentle yet effective way to manage weight amid this upheaval.

Greetings from a trip beyond the traditional paradigm of weight loss. This book is about more than just losing weight; it's about finding your body again, getting your energy back, and improving your connection to movement and yourself.

We will explore somatic exercises on these pages, which are a comprehensive approach to fitness that works the mind and muscles simultaneously. Somatic exercises offer a technique to achieve long-term weight loss and profound transformation by allowing us to explore the complex relationship between body and mind.

However, what are somatic exercises precisely, and how are they different from the plethora of modern fitness modalities? Somatic exercises focus on conscious movement and internal awareness. They are based on the principles of sensory-motor learning. Somatic exercises encourage us to tune into our bodies, listen to their wisdom, and move with intention and mindfulness, in contrast to standard workouts that frequently place a higher priority on external performance indicators.

your book provides a thorough explanation of somatic exercises and their significant impact on weight management, acting as your guide on your life-changing journey. Every chapter in this book, which covers everything from the subtleties of somatic movement techniques to the secrets of the mind-body connection, has been carefully designed to provide you with the information and resources you need to start your somatic weight reduction journey.

We allow the body's natural capacity for healing and transformation to be unlocked via posture correction, breathwork, and gentle movements. We can break free from the pattern of starvation and deprivation and adopt a holistic approach to health that nourishes the body, mind, and spirit by practicing awareness and present in our daily lives.

I encourage you to approach this journey with curiosity, openness, and compassion as you read through the pages that follow. Give up on the idea of quick solutions and trust the natural intelligence of your body. As we use the power of somatic exercises to unlock the vibrant, healthy, and joyful life that awaits us, let's set off on a journey of self-discovery together.

This book is more than simply a book; it's a path to emancipation, a voyage to become the whole version of ourselves. So, are you prepared to set out on this journey of transformation? Okay, let's get started.

## Understanding Somatic Exercises

When it comes to fitness and overall health, somatic exercises are a unique way to recognize and utilize the body's inherent intelligence. However, what are somatic exercises precisely, and how are they different from more conventional types of exercise?

Somatic exercises are fundamentally an integrative, attentive approach to movement and body awareness. In contrast to traditional exercise regimens that frequently concentrate only on outward performance and appearance, somatic exercises explore the deeper levels of proprioception, sensory-motor learning, and neuromuscular retraining.

Through the process of self-discovery, somatic exercises enable us to investigate the complex relationship that exists between our thoughts, emotions, and physical experiences. We develop a stronger feeling of presence and embodiment by learning to tune into the tiny cues of our bodies through mindfulness exercises, breathwork, and gentle movements.

The idea of "sensory-motor amnesia" is fundamental to the practice of somatic exercises. This is a condition in which past injuries, regular movement patterns, and long-term stress can leave some muscles tight or restricted. With the help of somatic exercises, stress patterns are released and ideal movement function is restored, promoting increased ease, flexibility, and vitality.

Furthermore, somatic exercises highlight how the neurological system controls muscle tension and coordination of movement. Through slow, intentional movement and somatic awareness practices, we retrain brain connections, improving proprioception and bringing the body-mind system back into harmony.

Somatic exercises, then, provide us with a means of reawakening the innate wisdom and resilience of our bodies. We become more aware of our physical capabilities and limitations through mindful movement and self-reflection, which enables us to move with grace, effectiveness, and energy.

## Somatic Movement's Benefits for Losing Weight

Many people ignore the holistic approach provided by somatic movement in favor of tight diets and rigorous exercise routines in their quest for weight loss. Somatic activities provide several advantages that go beyond weight loss and support long-term weight loss and general health.

1. Mind-Body Connection: Somatic movement places a strong emphasis on the connection between mind and body, encouraging a more profound understanding of how our feelings, ideas, and bodily experiences impact our interactions with food and exercise. Somatic activities foster presence and

mindfulness, which can assist people in developing more balanced food and movement habits and making healthier decisions.

2. Reduction of Stress: Prolonged stress is frequently linked to weight growth and trouble reducing weight. Somatic activities can reduce stress and foster a sense of peace and well-being by using breathing exercises, mindfulness exercises, and relaxation techniques. Somatic movement can help with emotional eating and promote weight loss goals by lowering stress levels.

3. Enhanced Kinesthetic Awareness and Proprioception: Somatic exercises improve proprioception and kinesthetic awareness, which helps people comprehend their bodies' signals and movement patterns. People can control their portion sizes and weight by paying attention to their hunger, fullness, and physical discomfort. This allows them to make better-educated decisions about what, when, and how much to eat.

4. Functional Movement Patterns: Somatic exercises encourage functional movement patterns that resemble everyday activities, in contrast to typical workouts that frequently concentrate on specific muscle groups or repeated motions. People gain strength, flexibility, and mobility through dynamic, multi-dimensional movement, which improves daily tasks and increases energy expenditure.

5. Postural Alignment and Core Strengthening: Somatic exercises focus on the deep core muscles that support and

stabilize the spine. People can reduce pressure on their spines, realign their bodies, and improve overall body symmetry by strengthening these muscles and correcting postural imbalances. This will result in a more functional and well-balanced body.

6. Long-Term Sustainability: Possibly most significantly, the somatic movement provides a long-term strategy for weight loss that emphasizes overall health and well-being. Somatic exercises help people establish lifelong habits and cognitive adjustments that support enduring transformation and continuing progress on their weight reduction journey, as opposed to focusing only on short-term results.

Essentially, somatic exercise has many advantages for weight loss that go much beyond physical changes. Somatic activities provide a holistic approach to long-term weight loss, increased energy, and improved general well-being by uniting the mind, body, and spirit.

# CHAPTER 1

# THE RELATIONSHIP BETWEEN THE MIND AND BODY

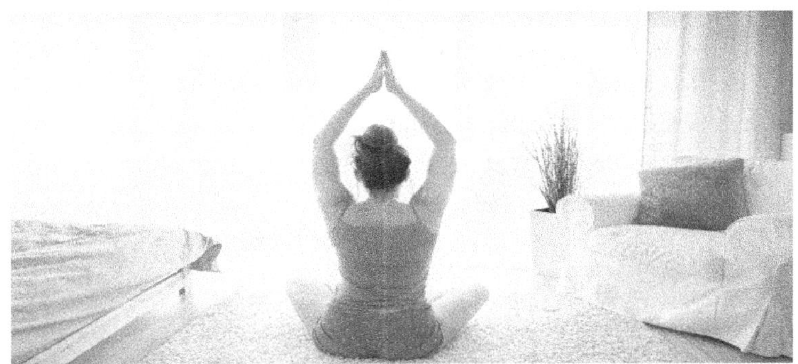

The foundation of somatic movement is the mind-body link, which also acts as a compass for comprehending the intricate relationship between our feelings, ideas, and bodily experiences. Examining this link in the context of weight loss provides priceless insights into the intricate processes that affect our relationship with food, activity, and body image.

The complex relationship between our mental and physical states is symbolized by the mind-body connection, which emphasizes how our attitudes, feelings, and ideas may affect how our bodies react to us and vice versa. To get long-lasting and comprehensive outcomes in the weight reduction context, it is critical to comprehend and investigate this relationship.

# Examining the Relationship Between Mind and Body in Weight Loss

**1. Stress and Its Impact**: Stress is a prevalent and ubiquitous aspect of contemporary life, and it has a significant impact on controlling weight. Stress causes our bodies to release hormones like cortisol, which can make us crave comfort foods that are heavy in calories. Furthermore, long-term stress can interfere with metabolism and encourage fat storage, which makes losing weight more difficult. Understanding how stress affects weight management, people can use stress-reduction strategies to lessen its effects and aid in their weight loss journey, such as deep breathing exercises, meditation, or somatic practices.

**2. Emotional Eating Patterns**: Our relationship with food is greatly influenced by our emotions, which frequently result in emotional eating patterns. Food can be a coping method used to distract or calm us when we are feeling stressed, depressed, bored, or other feelings. However doing so might lead to overindulging in unhealthy meals or overeating, which can undermine attempts to lose weight. People can create more balanced relationships with food and healthier coping mechanisms by investigating the emotional reasons behind these eating patterns and raising awareness of their emotions and hunger cues.

**3. Body Awareness and Healing:** Pain and suffering are frequently the result of emotional strain and trauma that our bodies are predisposed to storing. A comprehensive method for de-stressing, fostering healing, and reestablishing a connection with the body is provided by somatic exercises. People can improve body awareness and address underlying emotional issues that may be causing weight gain or difficulties decreasing weight by using gentle movements, breathwork, and mindfulness practices. People can support their weight reduction journey from a place of self-compassion and acceptance by developing a deeper connection with their bodies.

**4. Cognitive Shifts and Belief Systems:** Our self-perception and self-belief in our capacity for weight loss can have a significant impact on our actions and results. Self-sabotaging habits can be created by negative ideas like "I'll never be able to lose weight" or "I'm not worthy of being healthy," which can impede growth. A more positive relationship with oneself and one's body can be developed by questioning these ideas and embracing an attitude of self-compassion, empowerment, and possibilities. Affirmations, visualization methods, and cognitive reframing activities can assist people in changing their perspective and gaining more self-assurance that they can succeed in their weight loss objectives.

People can learn more about the intricate interactions between their ideas, feelings, and behaviors by investigating the mind-body connection in weight reduction. Through the integration of holistic well-being practices, such as somatic practices, emotional awareness exercises, stress reduction techniques, and mindset adjustments, people can have a transforming journey towards long-term weight loss and enhanced general health.

## How Somatic Exercises  Impact Body Awareness

It's very simple to lose touch with our bodies in the modern world when there are a lot of distractions and constant demands on our time. Amidst the commotion of everyday life, we could choose to ignore signs of exhaustion, push through pain, or simply forget to check in with ourselves. However, developing bodily awareness is crucial for general well-being, and somatic exercises provide an effective means of re-establishing this relationship.

A comprehensive method of movement, somatic exercises place a focus on inward awareness and conscious interaction with the body. Somatic techniques encourage us to tune into the subtle feelings and nuances of our physical experience, in contrast to traditional forms of exercise that only focus on aesthetics or external performance. We cultivate a stronger feeling of presence and embodiment by waking up to the rich tapestry of sensations that occupy our bodies via mindful practices, breathwork, and gentle movements.

However, in what precise way can somatic activities affect bodily awareness? Let's examine a few important mechanisms:

**1. Sensory-Motor Learning:** Through somatic exercises, we improve our sense, perception, and response to both internal and external stimuli. This process is known as sensory-motor learning. We can improve our proprioception, or the body's knowledge of its position in space, by consciously tuning into feelings like muscle tension, joint position, and breathing patterns. In addition to increasing movement efficiency and coordination, this increased proprioceptive awareness strengthens our bond with our bodies.

**2. Mindful Movement Practices:** The art of moving with conscious intention and attention to the present moment is a key component of somatic exercises. By moving slowly and deliberately, we develop a more acute awareness of our bodies and the feelings they generate. We learn to notice minute variations in our tense muscles, the cadence of our breathing, and the feel of our movements. By cultivating an embodied presence, this mindful method enables us to experience our bodies more fully and truthfully.

**3. Breath Awareness:** Breathwork functions as a link between the mind and body and is a crucial part of somatic exercises. We may establish a stronger connection to our bodies and ground ourselves in the present moment by focusing on the breath and its rhythm, depth, and quality. By focusing our attention inward and establishing a connection with our physical senses, conscious breathing not only helps us relax and reduce tension but also improves our awareness of our bodies.

**4. Release of Tension:** Somatic activities provide a mildly efficient way to relieve muscular tension and release tension. We address chronic tension areas by promoting relaxation and disentangling patterns of muscle holding with deliberate, methodical motions and mild stretching. We become more conscious of the minute changes in feeling that happen with relaxation as the tension releases, strengthening our bond with our bodies and encouraging an open and carefree attitude.

**5. Cultivation of Embodied Presence:** In the end, somatic practices help us develop our capacity for embodied presence, which is the capacity to occupy our bodies with awareness, compassion, and sincerity. By practicing these techniques, we develop the ability to pay attention to our bodies wisdom and respect their needs and boundaries. Knowing that our bodies are allies in the pursuit of health and completeness helps us to become more resilient and self-assured.

Somatic exercises provide a haven for reestablishing a connection with the wisdom of the body in a society that frequently pushes us to live in our minds. We reclaim our inheritance as sentient creatures capable of profound self-awareness and deep presence as we awaken to the richness of our embodied experience via mindful movement, breath awareness, and tension release. Now, as we rediscover the joy of being present in our bodies, let's set out on this voyage of inquiry and discovery.

# CHAPTER 2

## FUNDAMENTALS OF SOMATIC TRAINING

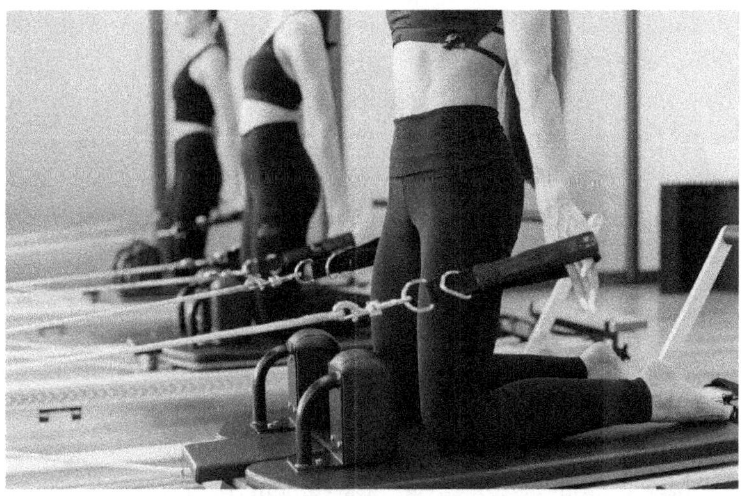

The fundamental ideas of somatic exercises serve as the cornerstone of an all-encompassing approach to movement and well-being. People can establish a more profound connection with their bodies and unleash the transforming power of somatic practices by comprehending and embodying these ideas.

## Fundamental Ideas in Somatic Movement

Several essential ideas that influence how we interact with our body and the environment around us serve as the foundation for somatic movement:

1. The technique of fully and deliberately inhabiting our bodies is known as embodied awareness, and it is the fundamental idea underlying somatic movement. A profound sense of presence and connection with our physical selves can be developed through somatic activities, as opposed to considering the body as a separate thing that can be managed or controlled. By paying conscious attention to our breath, movement, and sensations, we become more aware of the richness of our embodied experience and grow to value the wisdom that resides inside our bodies.

2. Sensory-Motor Learning: This theory, which highlights the crucial connection between sensory perception and motor control, is the foundation for somatic movement. Proprioception is improved, movement patterns are honed, and our comprehension of the capabilities and limitations of our bodies is expanded when we move slowly and deliberately and pay close attention to the sensory data that results from our actions. We can move with grace and ease because of the increased movement efficiency, coordination, and fluidity that this embodied learning process promotes.

3. Mindful Movement: Somatic movement is based on mindfulness, which helps us develop nonjudgmental acceptance of our body experience and present-moment

awareness. We learn to move with conscious intention, concentration, and curiosity through the practice of mindful movement. We also learn to tune into the subtleties and subtle sensations of our motions as they occur. We strengthen our connection to the world around us and ground ourselves in the present moment by focusing attention on the breath, the quality of movement, and the bodily sensations.

4. Dynamic Relaxation: Somatic movement places a strong emphasis on the value of dynamic relaxation, which is the skill of gently, non-forcefully releasing muscle-holding patterns and tension. Somatic exercises encourage us to participate in slow, exploratory movements that promote the release of tension and the restoration of natural movement patterns, as opposed to depending on external force or effort to stretch or strengthen muscles. We develop a sensation of comfort, suppleness, and relaxation in the body using techniques like pandiculation, mild rocking, and delicate articulations of the spine. This permits better mobility and increased energy.

5. Self-Exploration and Empowerment: In the end, somatic movement invites us to take an active role in our recovery and development by taking us on a path of self-exploration and empowerment. Somatic activities enable us to take charge of our health and well-being and to develop a deeper understanding of our bodies' needs and desires by promoting a sense of agency and self-efficacy. We regain our inherent ability to grow, be resilient, and heal ourselves via the process of self-expression and self-discovery, and we become fully realized as embodied beings.

One can access the transformative power of somatic practices and set out on a journey of profound self-discovery, healing, and personal growth by embodying these fundamentals of somatic movement: embodied awareness, sensory-motor learning, mindful movement, dynamic relaxation, and self-exploration and empowerment.

## Methods for Including Somatic Exercises in Everyday Activities

Even though somatic exercises are very beneficial for both physical and mental health, it might be difficult to fit them into your daily schedule with everything going on in today's hectic world. But it is possible and satisfying to incorporate somatic techniques into your daily life if you put in a little effort and are creative about it. The following strategies can assist you in incorporating somatic exercises into your daily schedule:

1. Mindful Movement Breaks: Throughout the day, take brief pauses to practice mindful movement. To relieve stress and encourage relaxation, try some mild stretching, deep breathing, or easy somatic exercises for a few minutes. Use these times to tune into your body and develop a sense of presence and well-being, whether you're at your desk, in the kitchen, or line.

2. Somatic Morning ritual: To create a great vibe for the day, begin your day with a somatic morning ritual. This could involve exercises like body scanning meditation, moderate yoga asanas, or mindful stretching to awaken your body, clear your mind, and get ready for the day. Your morning routine can be strengthened with somatic exercises, which help you cultivate mindfulness and self-care that will serve you well throughout the day.

3. Somatic Movement Snacks: Include somatic movement "snacks" in your everyday activities to avoid thinking of exercise as something you exclusively do at the gym or during set workout sessions. This could entail introducing mild motions into routine chores like dishwashing, folding laundry, or waiting for the kettle to boil, such as pelvic tilts, shoulder rolls, or spinal twists. Adding somatic exercises to your everyday routine turns menial tasks into chances for self-care, mindfulness, and movement.

4. Somatic Evening Wind-Down: To help you unwind and get ready for a good night's sleep, finish your day with a somatic evening ritual. To relieve stress, calm the mind, and encourage profound relaxation, try techniques like progressive muscle relaxation, gentle stretching, or guided meditation. You may tell your body and mind that it's time to relax and enter a state of rest and renewal by including somatic exercises in your nightly routine.

5. Mindful Movement Practices: Become aware of how you move and inhabit your body throughout the day to develop a mindful movement mindset. Whether you are moving, sitting,

standing, or performing an exercise, pay attention to your body's sensations, posture, and breathing. Identify any tight spots or uncomfortable spots, then use gentle motions or breathing exercises to relieve the tension. You can improve the advantages of somatic workouts and strengthen your relationship with your body by including awareness in your motions.

6. Incorporate Somatic Classes or Workshops: To enhance your practice and establish a supportive network of like-minded people, think about participating in somatic movement classes or workshops. Take part in group classes or seminars to get structure, direction, and inspiration to help you stick with your somatic practice, whether it's yoga, Feldenkrais, Alexander Technique, or another somatic discipline.

You can experience the health advantages of somatic exercises and develop a stronger bond with your body, mind, and spirit by incorporating these practices into your everyday routine. Whether it's through physical morning rituals, evening wind-down practices, or mindful movement breaks, discover ways to include moments of self-care, embodied awareness, and presence into your daily routine.

# CHAPTER 3

# WEIGHT LOSS AND BREATHWORK

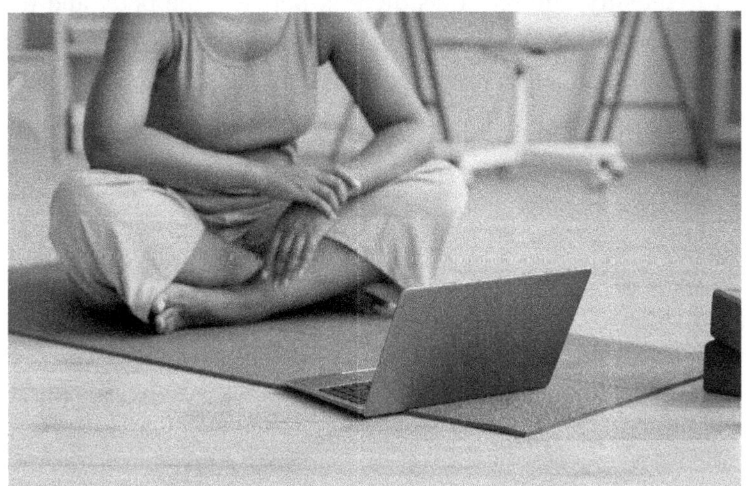

**B**reathwork is a key component of somatic practices; it can lead to improved health, lowered stress levels, and yes, even weight loss. Knowing the role that breath plays in somatic exercises will help us better understand how it affects our mental, emotional, and physical states.

## Breath: An Essential Part of Somatic Practices

Breath is a potent instrument for developing consciousness, balancing the nervous system, and encouraging relaxation. It is frequently referred to as the link between the body and the mind. Breathwork has various important functions in somatic activities that help with weight loss efforts:

1. Stress Reduction: Because chronic stress can lead to hormone imbalances, emotional eating, and cravings for unhealthy foods, it is frequently a barrier to weight loss. Breathwork methods that trigger the body's relaxation response, such as diaphragmatic breathing or deep belly breathing, help people relax by releasing tension, reducing cortisol levels, and fostering a peaceful frame of mind. Breathwork produces an ideal internal environment for weight loss by lowering tension and encouraging relaxation.

2. Mindful Eating: Mindful eating involves paying attention to the sensory experience of eating without judgment or distraction. A fundamental part of this practice is breath awareness. People can develop more awareness and present during mealtime rituals by integrating breathwork. This enables them to taste their food, pay attention to signals of hunger and fullness, and make more deliberate decisions about what and how much to eat. This increased awareness can help with portion control and weight management by preventing emotional eating, overeating, and mindless snacking.

3. Emotional Regulation: Breathwork is an effective technique for controlling cravings and emotions, two significant barriers to weight loss. Deep breathing exercises help people relax their nervous systems, quiet their minds, and make room for more intelligent reactions to emotional cues whether they are experiencing stress, anxiety, or food cravings. People can overcome emotional eating tendencies and create better-coping mechanisms for handling stress and unpleasant emotions by increasing their emotional resilience and self-awareness through breathwork.

4. Enhanced Metabolism: The parasympathetic nerve system, which regulates digestion, rest, and relaxation, can be activated with deep breathing exercises. Breathwork facilitates proper digestion and metabolism by inducing the parasympathetic response, which enhances the body's ability to burn calories and absorb nutrients from food. Deep breathing exercises also help general metabolic function and vitality by increasing circulation, boosting energy levels, and improving blood oxygenation.

5. Body Awareness: Breathwork offers a direct route to the interior terrain of the body by acting as a link between the aware and unconscious parts of the mind. People can become more aware of their bodies and acquire somatic intelligence by learning to tune into the rhythm, depth, and quality of their breath. This will enable them to recognize subtle cues such as physical discomfort, satiety, and hunger. This increased awareness can support long-term weight loss and general well-being by empowering people to make better decisions about their diet, exercise routine, and self-care routines.

Breathwork is essentially a fundamental component of somatic activities that has significant advantages for both holistic health and weight loss. People can use the transforming power of the breath to assist their weight reduction objectives, develop better self-awareness, and improve their overall quality of life by implementing breath awareness, deep breathing methods, and mindful breathing activities into their daily lives.

## Breathing Techniques for Relaxation and Stress Reduction

Stress has become a regular companion for many in our fast-paced world, negatively impacting our physical and mental health. But even in the middle of all the craziness, the act of breathing itself provides a potent tool for stress relief and relaxation. You can use the calming power of the breath to encourage resilience, balance, and a sense of serenity by implementing certain breathing exercises into your daily routine. The following are some efficient breathing methods for relieving tension and promoting relaxation:

1. Deep belly breathing, or diaphragmatic breathing:
By activating the diaphragm muscle, diaphragmatic breathing is a straightforward but effective method for reducing tension and fostering calm. For diaphragmatic breathing exercises:

- Find a sitting or laying position that is comfortable.
- Put your hands on your abdomen and your chest, respectively.
- Take a deep breath through your nose, feeling your abdomen lift as air enters your lungs.
- Breathe out slowly through your lips while allowing your belly to drop slightly.
- For several minutes, keep up this deep, rhythmic breathing pattern, paying attention to how your breath enters and exits your body.

2. Square breathing, or box breathing:
Box breathing is a method of controlled breathing in which you aim to equalize the length of your breaths and the intervals between them. This technique aids in nervous system regulation and calmness promotion. To work on breathing in a box:

- Take a deep breath through your nose and hold it for four seconds to fill your lungs up entirely.
- For four counts, hold your breath at the peak of the inhale while keeping your body relaxed and spacious.
- Release tension and stress with each breath by gently and fully exhaling through your mouth for four counts.
- As you prepare to start the next breath cycle, hold your breath at the bottom of the exhale for four seconds.
- Continue in this manner for a few rounds, extending the duration of each breath cycle as you get more accustomed to the technique.

3. Breathing (Calm Breath) in 4-7-8:
Dr. Andrew Weil developed the 4-7-8 breathing technique, which is a straightforward yet powerful way to induce relaxation and lower stress levels. To engage in 4-7-8 breathing exercises:

- To start, release all of the tension in your body by fully exhaling through your mouth and creating a whooshing sound.
- Shut your mouth and take four slow, quiet breaths through your nose, letting your belly swell with each one.
- While holding your breath at the peak of the inhalation, keep your body steady and tranquil for seven seconds.
- Breathe out gently and fully through your mouth for eight seconds, letting go of any last bits of tension.
- Breathe in this manner four times, concentrating on the feeling of calm with each exhale.

4. Nadi Shodhana, or Alternate Nostril Breathing:
An ancient yogic practice, alternate nostril breathing relaxes the mind and balances the body's energy flow. To practice breathing through different noses:

- Take a comfortable seat with your shoulders back and your spine straight.
- Seal your right nostril with your thumb, then take a four-second deep breath through your left nostril.
- Seal your left nostril with your right ring finger, then hold your breath for four seconds.
- Let go of your right thumb and take a slow, four-second breath out of your right nostril.

- Take a deep inhale into your right nostril for four counts. Then, shut it with your thumb and hold your breath for another four counts.
- Let go of your left ring finger and take a slow, four-second breath out of your left nostril.
- Breathe in this alternate pattern for multiple rounds, noticing the balancing and relaxing benefits as you go.

By incorporating these breathing techniques into your daily routine, you can both foster a better sense of relaxation and well-being over time and receive immediate relief from stress and anxiety. The power of breath is a straightforward yet effective technique that may be used alone or in conjunction with other mindfulness exercises like yoga or meditation to achieve inner calm and resilience in the face of adversity.

# CHAPTER 4

# SOMATIC ACTIVITIES TO INCREASE FLEXIBILITY AND MOBILITY

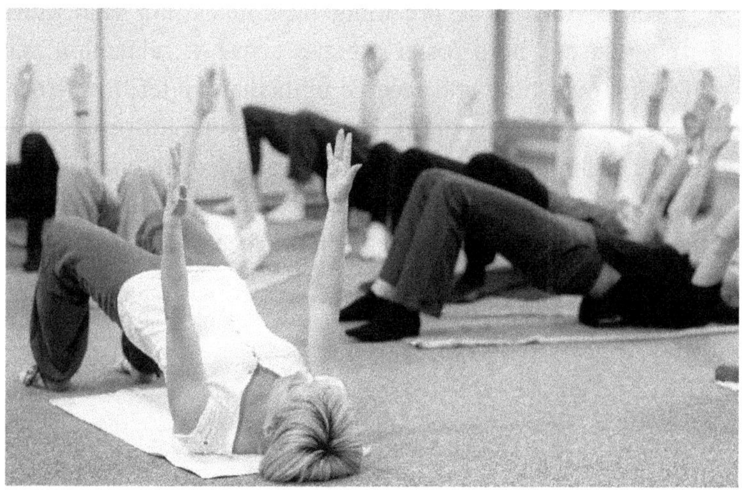

Somatic exercises provide a mild yet efficient method for increasing joint flexibility and mobility, enabling people to move with more grace, ease, and fluidity. Somatic exercises improve the range of motion, reduce joint stiffness, and retrain the neuromuscular system by releasing patterns of muscular tension and improving mobility. To increase joint mobility through somatic practices, try these mild movements:

# Mild Motions to Enhance Joint Flexibility

**1. Shoulder Rolls:**

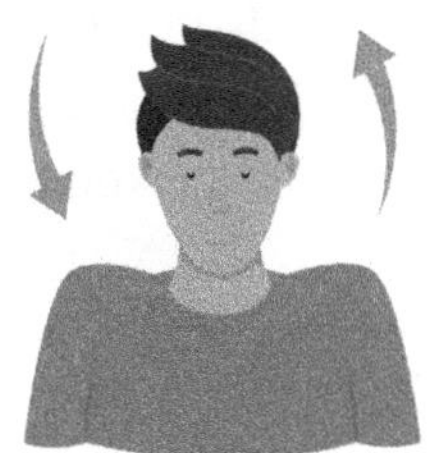

- Take a comfortable seat or stand with your shoulders back and your spine straight.

- As you slowly bring your chin up to your chest, you should feel a slight stretch in the nape of your neck.

As you start to turn your head to the right, your right ear will move closer to your right shoulder.

- Keep moving in a circular manner, rolling your head to the left and putting your left ear up to your left shoulder before returning it to the center.

- Perform numerous rounds of this circular motion, paying attention to your movements and letting your breath direct them.

- To explore your neck's whole range of motion, reverse the direction of the circles.

**2. Chest of Shoulders:**

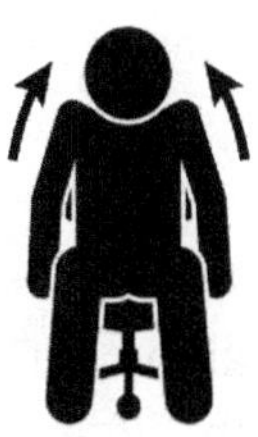

- Place your feet hip-width apart and keep your arms at your sides in a relaxed manner.

- Take a breath and raise your shoulders to your ears, pulling them back.

Squeeze your shoulder blades together and release

the breath as you move your shoulders back and down.
- Keep moving in this circular motion, breathing in as you raise and lower your shoulders and out as you roll them back and forth.

- To explore other shoulder angles and ranges of motion, reverse the direction of the circles.
- Continue doing this for a few rounds, moving easily and letting your breathing direct your movements.

**3. Cervical Waves:**
- Place your feet hip-width apart and bend your knees just a little bit.
- For support, rest your hands on your hips or the small of your back.
- Take a breath, raise your chest and push your pelvis forward while arching your spine.
- Tuck your chin into your chest and tilt your pelvis back as you release the breath as you round your spine.
- Keep doing this flowing movement, gracefully transitioning with each breath from a backbend to a forward fold.
- Explore your spine's whole range of motion by letting the movement flow naturally with your breath.
- Repeat multiple times, paying attention to how your spine feels like it's stretching and opening.

## 4. Circles of Hip:

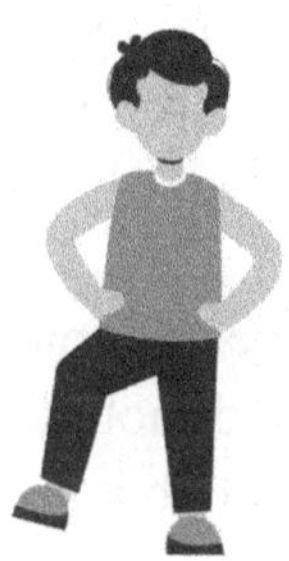

- Place your hands on your hips for support and stand with your feet hip-width apart.
- Breathe in as you raise your right knee to your chest and make clockwise circles with it.
- Release the breath as you bring your right foot back to the floor and move to your left leg, doing counterclockwise circles with your left knee.
- Maintain this circular movement, switching your breathing between your left and right legs.
- Pay attention to keeping your supporting leg stable and letting your hip joint move naturally.

- Continue for multiple rounds, experimenting with circle sizes and speeds to increase hip joint mobility.

## 5. Crowns on the ankle:

- With your feet flat on the floor, choose a comfortable seat or stand.
- Raising your right foot off the ground, start drawing clockwise circles with your right ankle.
- Concentrate on extending your ankle's range of motion and using your toes to make wide circles.
- After a few rounds, transfer to your left foot and make counterclockwise circles with your left ankle.
- Keep moving in a circular manner, switching between your left and right ankles with each breath.
- Be attentive to any regions that feel stiff or resistant, and explore them

gently while maintaining
awareness.

- Continue for a few
cycles, letting your ankles
relax and release tension
as you go.

These mild somatic exercises provide a comprehensive
method for increasing joint flexibility and mobility, enabling
people to move more freely and comfortably in their own
bodies. Through the integration of these movements into your
everyday regimen and the practice of mindful awareness, you
can improve the flexibility and health of your joints, lessen
pain and stiffness, and develop a stronger sense of body
awareness.

# Stretching Patterns to Increase Flexibility

Being flexible is essential for maintaining general physical health and well-being because it increases movement, lowers the chance of injury, and improves athletic performance. Stretching exercises can improve flexibility, release tense muscles, and encourage relaxation when incorporated into your regimen. The following are some efficient stretching exercises to increase flexibility:

## 1. The Whole-Body Stretching Sequence:

This exercise routine promotes general flexibility and mobility by focusing on the body's key muscle groups.

### 1. Finding a Forward Position:
- Place your feet hip-width apart when standing.
- Take a breath and extend your spine by raising your arms above your head.
- Let out a breath as you bend forward and hinge at the hips, reaching your hands to your shins or the ground.
- Let your head hang heavy and relax your shoulders and neck.
- Hold the position for 30 to 60 seconds while taking deep breaths into the stretch.

### 2. Dog Facing Downward:

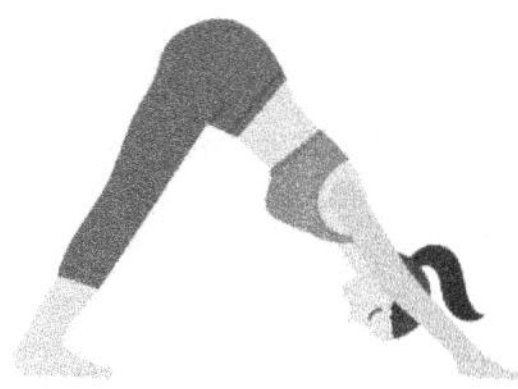

- Begin in the tabletop position, hands and knees together.

- Form an inverted V with your hips by pressing into your hands and lifting them up and back.
- Maintain a slight bend in your knees and extend your heels toward the floor.
- Extend your spine through your chest and press it toward your thighs.
- Breathe deeply, hold for 30 to 1 minute, and concentrate on opening your shoulders and lengthening your spine.

**3. Deep Breath:**
- Step your right foot forward between your hands while in a downward-facing dog.
- Untuck your toes and drop your left knee to the floor.
- Slump your hips down and forward until your left hip feels stretched.
- Maintain a long spine and a raised chest.
- Switch sides after 30 to 1 minute of holding.

## 4. Front-facing Seat:

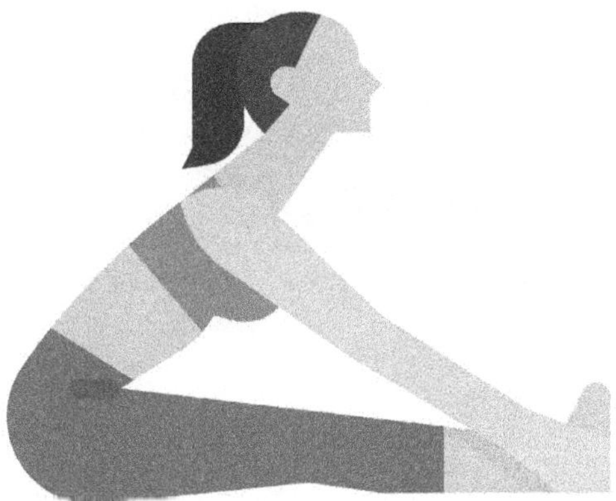

- Extend your legs in front of you while sitting on the ground.
- Take a breath and raise your arms above your head while lengthening your spine.
- Release the breath as you bend forward, extending your hips to grab your shins or feet.
- Maintain an open chest and a flat back.
- Breathe deeply and give in to the stretch as you hold for 30 to 1 minute.

## 5. Crow Pose:

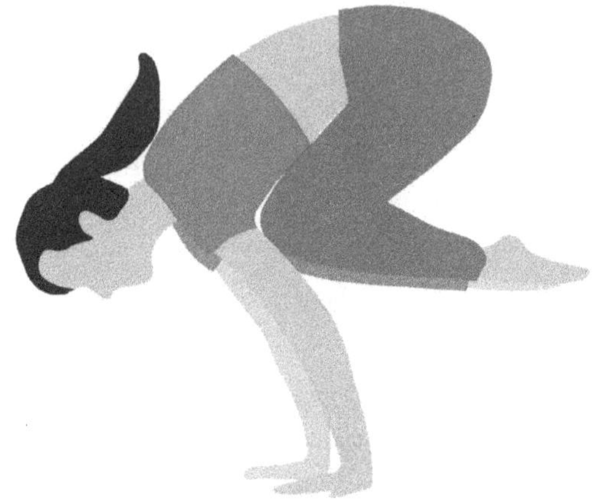

- While sitting, move your right foot to your left wrist and your right knee to your right wrist.
- With your hips positioned squarely in front of the mat, extend your left leg behind you.
Feel the stretch in your right hip and glute as you lower your hips toward the floor.
For a more thorough stretch, you can choose to fold forward over your right shin.
- Switch sides after 30 to 1 minute of holding.

## 2. Stretching Sequence for Upper Body:

Stretching the muscles of the upper body, such as the shoulders, chest, and back, is the main goal of this exercise.

### 1. Side Stretch and Child's Pose:

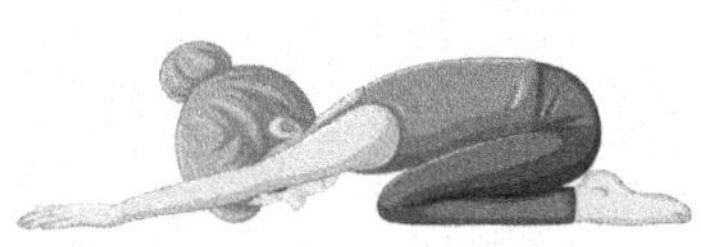

- Begin by placing your toes together and your knees apart while kneeling.
- Lower your chest toward the floor while sitting back on your heels and extending your arms forward.
- Feel the left side of your body extend as you walk your hands to the right.
- Switch sides after 30 to 1 minute of holding.

### 2. Thread the needle:

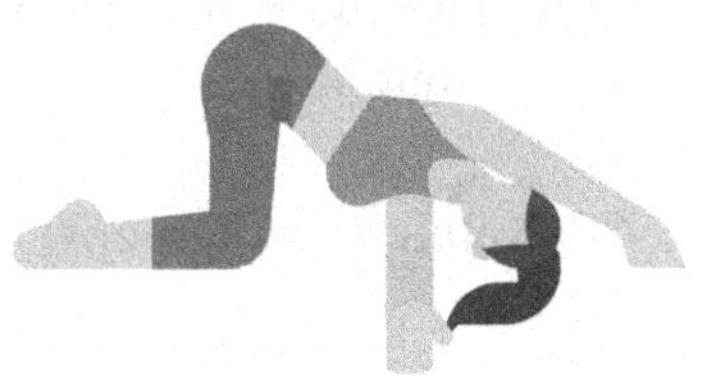

Place yourself on your hands and knees like you're on a table.
- Thread the needle by reaching your right arm under your left arm.
- Feel the stretch in your upper back and right shoulder as you lower your ear and shoulder to the floor.
- Switch sides after 30 to 1 minute of holding.

**3. Handheld Chest Wiper:**

- Arrange your arms behind you and place your feet hip-width apart.
- With your hands clasped together, slowly raise your arms to open your shoulders and chest.
Maintain a long spine and relaxed shoulders.
- Hold the position for 30 to 60 seconds while taking deep breaths into the stretch.

**4. Stretch Your Triceps:**

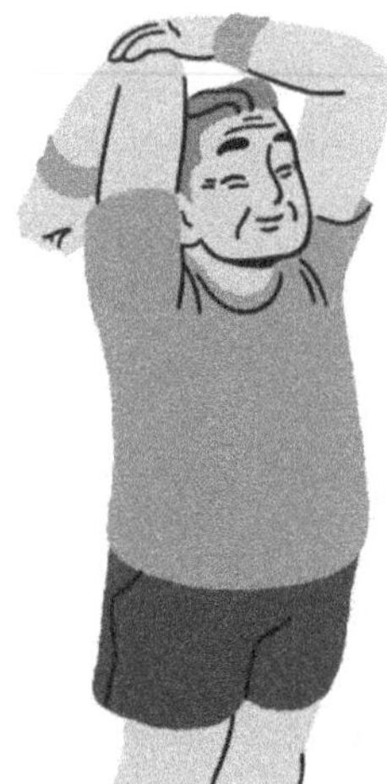

Bend your elbow and raise your right arm above, bringing your right hand to the middle of your upper back.
- To increase the stretch in your right triceps, lightly press with your left hand on your right elbow.
- Maintain an open chest and loose shoulders.
- Switch sides after 30 to 1 minute of holding.

**5. Extend Your Shoulders:**

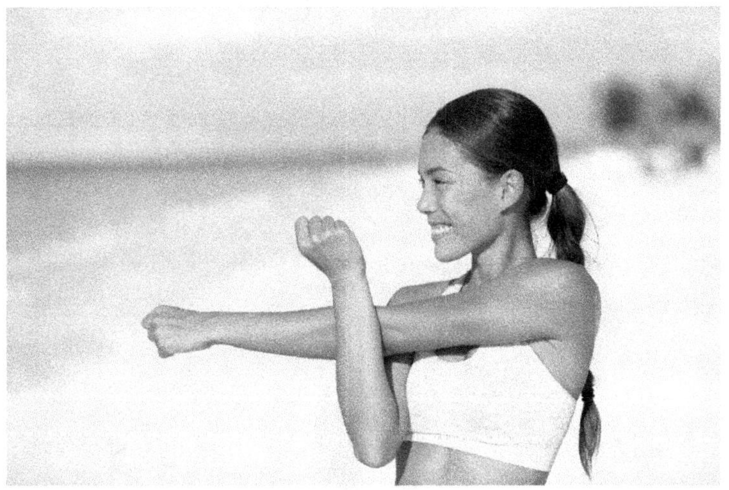

- Raise your right arm to shoulder height and spread it across your body.
- To bring your right arm closer to your chest, lightly press on your right elbow with your left hand.
Keep your spine straight and your shoulders relaxed.
- Switch sides after 30 to 1 minute of holding.

Include these stretching exercises in your regimen to increase your range of motion, lessen tense muscles, and enhance general health. Always pay attention to your body's needs and take deep breaths during each stretch to let go of any tension and find comfort in the motion.

# CHAPTER 5

## RELEASING STRESS AND TENSION

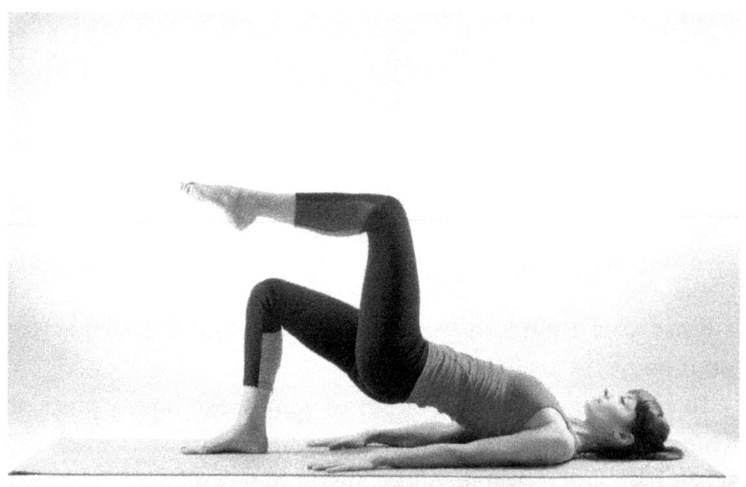

Stress negatively impacts our physical, mental, and emotional health and has become an inescapable aspect of modern life. By addressing both the underlying mental strain and the physical signs of stress in the body, somatic therapies provide a comprehensive approach to stress reduction. You can alleviate stress, encourage calmness, and develop more resilience by implementing somatic techniques into your everyday routine. Here are a few somatic methods for lowering stress:

# Physical Methods to Reduce Stress

**1. Meditation using Body Scan:**

- Close your eyes while you're sitting or lying down in a comfortable position.
- Start by focusing on your breath and allowing it to slow down and become deeper.
- Focus on every part of your body, beginning at your feet, and feel for any spots where you could be tense or uncomfortable.
- As you locate tense spots, intentionally relax and soften the corresponding muscles to allow them to loosen up.
- Keep looking over your body, focusing on your arms, shoulders, neck, head, legs, hips, abdomen, and chest as you move higher.
- Focus on each place for a short while while taking deep breaths and promoting calm and relaxation.
- Return to your breathing while experiencing a sensation of spaciousness and calmness throughout your body and mind to finish the body scan.

**2. Standardization:**

- To reset the length of the muscles at rest, a natural movement pattern called parasthesis entails slowly contracting and releasing the muscles.
- To start, tense a particular muscle group, like your back, shoulders, or neck, very lightly.
- After a few seconds of holding the contraction, gradually release the tension to allow the

muscles to extend and relax.
- Repeat this procedure multiple times, progressively becoming more conscious of your body's sensations and the minute variations in tense muscles.

- Pay close attention to the movement's quality, moving deliberately and slowly to completely participate in the pandiculation process.
- Take note of how pandiculating makes your body feel, and savor the sensation of relief and calm that ensues.

**3. Regulation and Awareness of Breath:**
- One of the most effective methods for lowering tension and relaxing the neurological system is deep breathing.
- Take a seat comfortably, then close your eyes.
Start paying attention to your breathing and the rhythm of your natural intake and release.
- Breathe in deeply through your nose, then out slowly through your mouth, gradually lengthening and deepening it.
- With each breath, feel the rise and fall of your belly with one hand, highlighting the expansion and contraction of your diaphragm.
As you continue to breathe deeply, feel the relaxation and calmness spread throughout your body. Let go of any tension or stress with each exhale.
Spend a few minutes using this breath awareness and control technique, letting each breath take you farther and deeper into a relaxed state.

## 4. Calm Motion and Light Stretching:

- Stretching exercises and moderate movement can reduce physical stress and encourage relaxation.
- Select a few basic exercises, including neck stretches, shoulder rolls, or mild spinal twists.
- Move carefully and slowly, focusing on your body's sensations and any tight or uncomfortable spots.

Breathe deeply into the stretch as you perform it, letting your breath direct your movements and help you release tension.
- Move in a way that feels supportive and nutritious to your body, putting more emphasis on the quality of the movement than the quantity.
- After finishing your stretching exercise, pause and observe how your body feels. Savor the sensation of ease and calm that arises from attentive movement.

## 5. Imagery and Visualization:

- One of the most effective methods for lowering tension and encouraging relaxation is visualization.
- Look for a peaceful, cozy area where you can sit or lie down.
- To center yourself, close your eyes and inhale deeply several times.
- Start by mentally picturing a calm and pleasant location, such as a placid beach, a lush forest, or a beautiful garden.
- Immerse yourself in the visualization by using all of your senses to picture the sights, sounds, smells, and sensations of this tranquil location.
- Give yourself permission to sink completely into the visualization, experiencing a wave of peace and quiet.

- Take in the sensations of calm and relaxation by spending as much time as feels comfortable in this visualization.

By incorporating these somatic practices into your everyday routine, you can alleviate tension, lower your stress level, and develop a more tranquil and well-being mindset. These methods, which can be used separately or in conjunction with one another to create a thorough stress-reduction regimen, are helpful for encouraging calmness and fortitude in the face of adversity.

## Using Somatic Practices to Address Emotional Eating

Emotional eating, or the propensity to use food as a comfort, a way to decompress, or a diversion from uncomfortable feelings, can have a negative impact on one's emotional and physical health. By encouraging a closer relationship with the body, developing self-awareness, and offering substitute coping mechanisms for handling emotions, somatic activities provide a comprehensive solution to the problem of emotional eating. The following somatic methods can be used to treat emotional eating:

1. Mindful Eating and Body Awareness:
- Cultivating awareness of physical sensations, such as cues related to hunger and satisfaction, is emphasized by somatic activities.

Spend a few minutes checking in with your body before eating. Take note of any bodily feelings you may have, such as stress, hunger, or fullness.

- Eat with awareness, focusing on the flavor, texture, and scent of your food. Chew gently, enjoying every taste.

- Pay attention to how your body reacts to certain foods. Do you find that some foods fill you up and give you energy, while others make you feel uncomfortable or lethargic?

- You can have a healthier connection with food and lessen the need to eat in reaction to emotional triggers by paying attention to your body's signals and meeting its requirements.

2. Relaxation Techniques and Breathwork:
Stress, anxiety, and other challenging emotions are frequently the cause of emotional eating. Relaxation and nervous system regulation are two benefits of somatic breathwork.

Engage in deep breathing techniques to help relax your body and mind. Breathe gently out through your mouth, letting go of tension and stress with each breath. Take a deep breath through your nose to fill your lungs with air.

- Use breathwork as a technique to instantly manage emotional distress. Instead of giving in to the temptation to overeat when you're stressed, take a few deep breaths. Take note of your body's reaction and any shifts in your mental state.

- You may lessen your tendency to turn to food for comfort and increase your resilience to stress by implementing breathwork into your daily routine.

3. Body Language and Motion:
- Somatic movement techniques provide a means of expressing and letting go of emotions that are held inside the body.
- Practice mild movement techniques to relieve physical stress and enhance emotional health, such as yoga, dance, or qigong.
- Give yourself permission to move in an instinctive manner, respecting your body's individual needs and expressions as it moves naturally.
- Pay attention to any feelings that surface while moving. Without passing judgment or criticizing yourself, give yourself permission to completely feel and express these feelings.
- You can release emotional energy held in your body and lessen the need to eat to cope with challenging emotions by mindfully and expressively moving your body.

4. Body-Mind Harmony:
- Somatic activities cultivate a sense of wholeness and connection by connecting the mind and body.
- Practice body-centered mindfulness techniques to increase your awareness of the mind-body link, such as progressive muscle relaxation, body scans, or guided imagery.
- Take note of how emotions cause physical feelings in the body. Are there any spots of stress, pain, or numbness associated with certain feelings?
- Develop an attitude of acceptance and self-compassion toward your body and its feelings. Allow yourself to fully feel your emotions with love and curiosity, rather than passing judgment or repressing them.

- You may create healthier coping mechanisms for handling emotions and lessen your dependency on food as your main emotional regulation tool by developing a stronger sense of body-mind integration.

5. Developing Self-Compassion
- Emotional eating is frequently accompanied by self-criticism, guilt, or humiliation. Somatic exercises can support the development of acceptance and self-compassion for oneself and one's experiences.
Engage in self-compassion exercises or loving-kindness meditation to develop acceptance, love, and kindness toward yourself.
- If you find yourself feeling the need to eat because of challenging feelings, take a moment to console and uplift yourself. Remind yourself that you are not alone in your struggles with emotional eating; it is a common human experience.
- Be nice and understanding to yourself as you would a friend going through a similar experience. Realize that you are doing the best you can with the tools at your disposal and that emotional eating is a coping technique rather than a character's fault.
- You can build a more supportive and loving environment within yourself by practicing self-compassion, which will lessen the need to turn to food for solace or approval.

You can manage emotional eating and develop a better relationship with food and your body by including somatic activities in your routine. A comprehensive strategy for mending the mind-body connection and advancing emotional well-being is provided by somatic practices, which cultivate increased self-awareness, emotional regulation, and the development of substitute coping mechanisms.

# CHAPTER 6

## SOMATIC EXERCISES FOR STRENGTHENING THE CORE

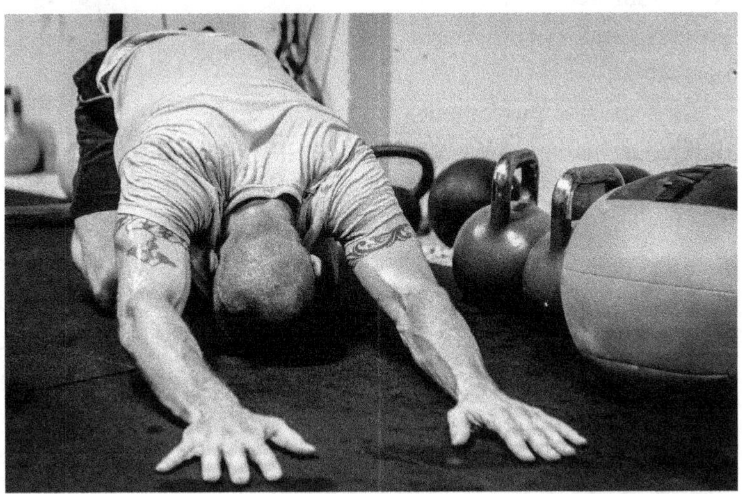

Posture, balance, and general stability all depend on a robust core. Somatic exercises are a mild yet efficient way to build stronger core muscles, which leads to increased resilience and more functional movement. Somatic exercises help develop strength from the inside out by actively and consciously using the core muscles, which promotes a strong bond between the body and mind. Here are some somatic exercises for strengthening the core:

### 1. Pelvic tilts:

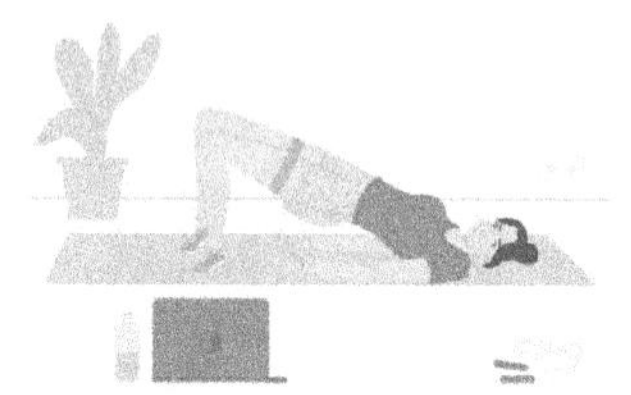

- Lay flat on your back with your feet flat on the ground and your knees bent.
- To feel the movement, put your hands on your pelvis.
- Take a preparatory breath, then release it as you flatten your lower back into the floor by tilting your pelvis towards your navel.
- Take a breath to bring your body back to neutral and restore your lower back's natural arch.
- Carry out multiple repetitions of this exercise, syncing it with your breathing.
- Pay close attention to using your transverse abdominis and other deep core muscles, as well as keeping your spine and pelvis stable.

### 2. Supine Leg slide:

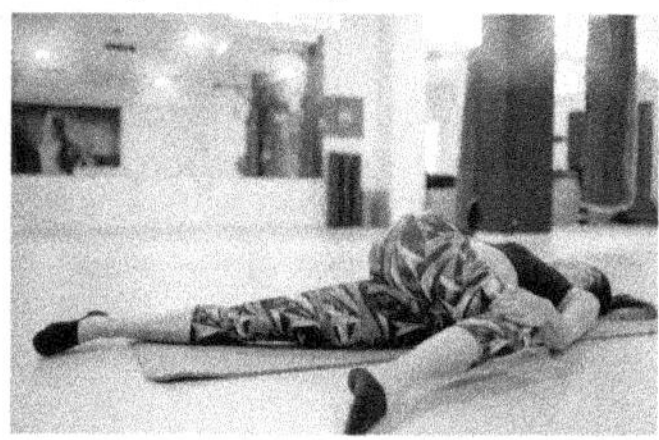

- Lay flat on your back with your feet flat on the ground and your knees bent.
- Take a breath to warm up, then release it as you move one foot away from your body and straighten your leg on the ground.
- Take a breath to bring the foot back to its initial position.
- Repeat many times on the opposite side, switching between the legs.
- Avoid any lower back twisting or arching by maintaining a solid pelvis

and an active core throughout the exercise.

## 3. Dead Bugs:

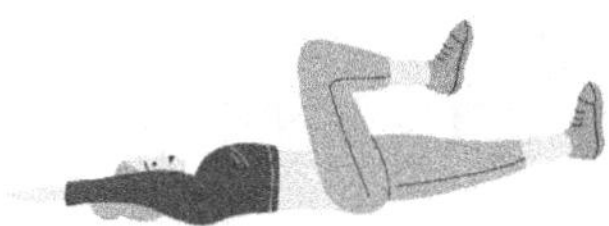

- Lay flat on your back with your knees bent 90 degrees and your arms extended toward the ceiling.
- Take a breath to warm up, then release it as you raise your right arm overhead and erect your left leg toward the ground.
- Take a breath to bring yourself back to the beginning position. Then, repeat on the opposite side, lifting your left arm overhead and bringing your right leg straight down toward the floor.
- Keep switching sides and repeat the action numerous times while syncing it with your breathing.
- Pay close attention to keeping your pelvis and core stable; avoid bending or shifting your lower back.

## 4. Spinal Twist in Sitting:

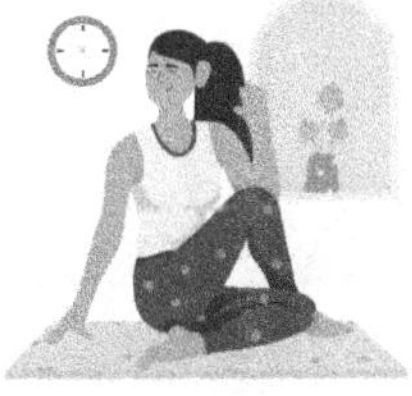

- Extend your legs in front of you while sitting on the floor.
- Place your right foot on the floor outside of your left knee, bending your right knee and crossing it over your left thigh.
- Breathe in to stretch your spine; exhale as you rotate to the right, landing your right hand on the floor behind you and your left elbow on the outside of your right knee.

- Breathe in to extend your spine even farther, and out as you twist more deeply, turning your torso to the right with a gentle exhale.

- Feel the stretch in your side body and spine as you hold the twist for a few breaths.
- Breathe in to center yourself again, and then do the opposite side.

## 5. Opposite quadruple arm and leg lift:

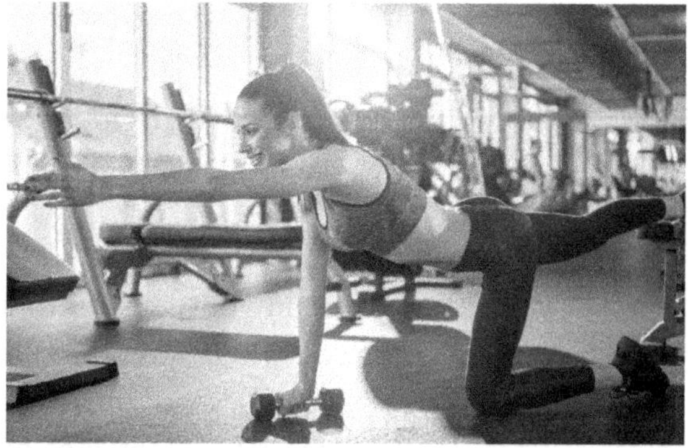

- Assume a tabletop position on your hands and knees, placing your knees behind your hips and your wrists beneath your shoulders.
- Breathe in to get ready, then release as you bring your left leg back and your right arm forward, parallel to the ground.
- Take a breath to bring yourself back to the beginning position. Then, repeat on the opposite side, extending your right leg back and your left arm forward.
- Keep switching sides and repeat the action numerous times while syncing it with your breathing.
- Avoid any lower back arching or rounding by concentrating on keeping your pelvis and core stable.

## 6. Bridge Pose

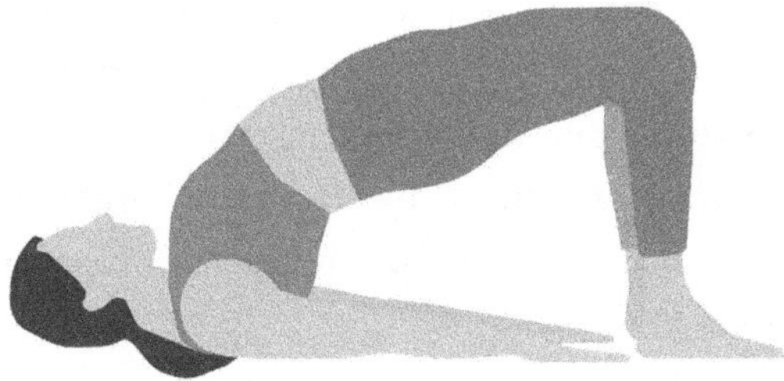

- Lay flat on your back with your feet hip-width apart and your knees bent.
- Breathe in to get ready, then release as you press your feet into the ground and raise your hips toward the ceiling.
- To support your pelvis and lower back, contract your glutes and core muscles.
- Stay in the bridge pose for a few breaths, focusing on your lower body and core stability and strength.
- Breathe in to controllably bring your hips back down to the floor.
- Carry out multiple repetitions, synchronizing the motion with your breathing.

You can include these somatic exercises for strengthening your core to your routine to help you become more resilient, strong, and stable. By using your core muscles consciously and deliberately, you may create a solid foundation for your general mobility and well-being. As usual, pay attention to your body and adjust the workouts to your own needs and capabilities.

## Abdominal Toning and Sculpting Exercises

In addition to being physically beautiful, a toned and sculpted abdomen is essential for overall core strength and stability. You can improve posture and functional movement while achieving your intended outcomes by including focused exercises in your program. The following are some efficient belly toning and shaping exercises:

### 1. Bicycle Crunches

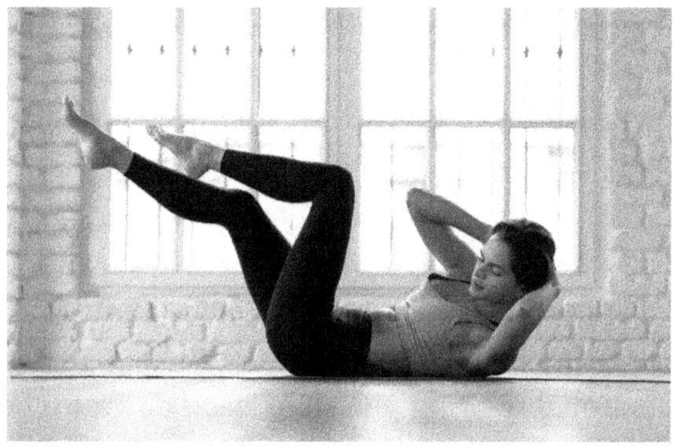

- While lying on your back, raise your legs and bend your knees to a 90-degree angle. Place your hands behind your head.
- Lift your shoulder blades off the ground by using your core muscles.
- While keeping your right leg straight, bend your right elbow toward your left knee.
- Switch sides, straightening your left leg and bringing your left elbow up to your right knee.

- Keep cycling in an alternate manner from side to side while concentrating on twisting from your core and maintaining control over your actions.

## 2. Variations in Planks:

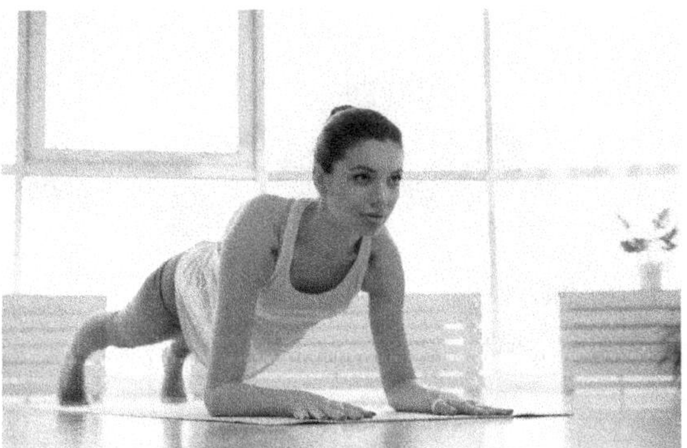

- Standard Plank: Place your hands directly under your shoulders and align your body in a straight line from your head to your heels to start. Hold while using your core and maintaining a level hip flexion for 30 to 1 minute.
- Side Plank: Place your feet on top of each other while lying on your side with your legs extended. Elevate your hips off the ground and rely on your forearm and bottom foot to sustain your weight. Hold each side for 30 to 1 minute, keeping your body in a straight line from your head to your heels.
- Plank with Knee Tucks: Begin in the familiar plank pose. Using your obliques, bring your right knee near your right elbow. Go back to the beginning and carry out the same action on the left side. Repeat alternate sides for ten to fifteen repetitions.

## 3. Russian Twist:

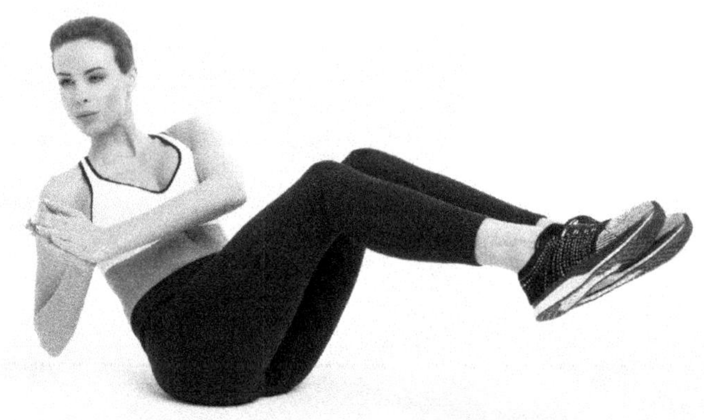

- Bend your knees and place your feet flat on the floor while you sit on the floor. Maintain a straight back while bending gently.
- To increase resistance, clench your fists together in front of your chest or grip a weight.
- Raise your feet off the floor and maintain your sit bones for balance.
- Turn your body to the right and bring your weight or clasped hands to the ground near your right hip.
Once you're back in the center, rotate to the left and shift your weight or hands to the floor in front of your left hip.
- Keep switching sides for ten to fifteen reps on each side, making sure to contract your obliques with each twist.

## 4. Leg Lifts:

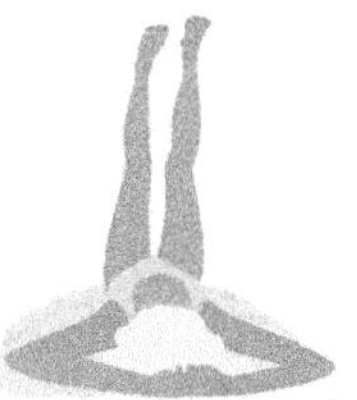

- Lay flat on your back with your arms at your sides and your legs straight.
- Lift your legs straight up toward the ceiling by using your core muscles.
- Lower your legs gradually toward the floor, stopping just short of making contact with the floor.
Raise your legs back to the beginning posture. Focus on deliberate motions and maintain your lower back pressed into the floor while you perform the exercise ten to fifteen times.

## 5. Mountain Ascentionists:

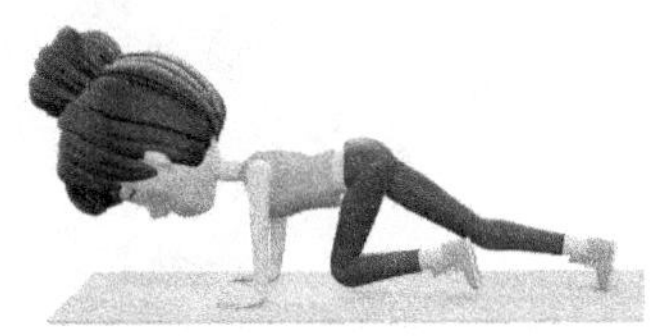

- Begin in the plank position, keeping your body in a straight line and your hands directly beneath your shoulders.
- Using your core, quickly switch legs and bring your left knee to your chest. - Next, move your right knee towards your chest.
- Keep sprinting with your legs alternately, moving quickly while keeping your plank form correct.
- Do mountain climbers for 30 to 1 minute, paying close attention to maintaining a strong core and solid hips.

### 6. V-Ups:

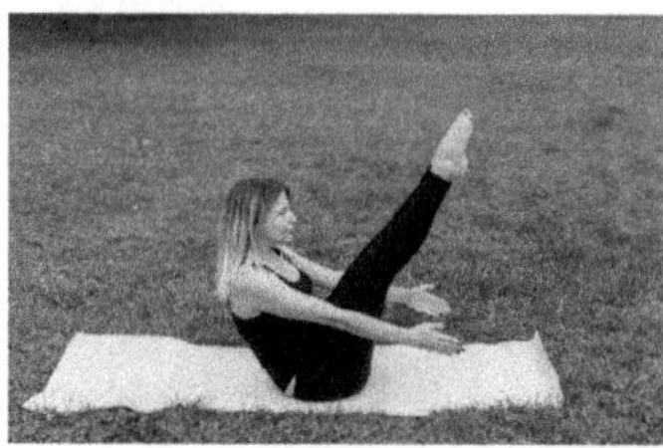

- While lying on your back, raise your arms upward and keep your legs straight.
- Using your core, raise your upper body and legs off the ground. Reach your hands down to your toes to create a V-shaped formation with your body.
- Controlfully descend back to the starting position slowly.
- Focus on lifting from your core and keeping your balance throughout the exercise as you perform the same 10 to 15 times.

Include these workouts in your regimen two to three times a week, escalating the difficulty and number of repetitions as your strength and endurance improve. To optimize performance and reduce the chance of injury, never forget to concentrate on good form and technique. Incorporating cardiovascular activity and maintaining a healthy diet into your overall fitness regimen will also assist in toning and shaping the abdomen area.

# CHAPTER 7

# ADJUSTING POSTURE TO LOSE WEIGHT

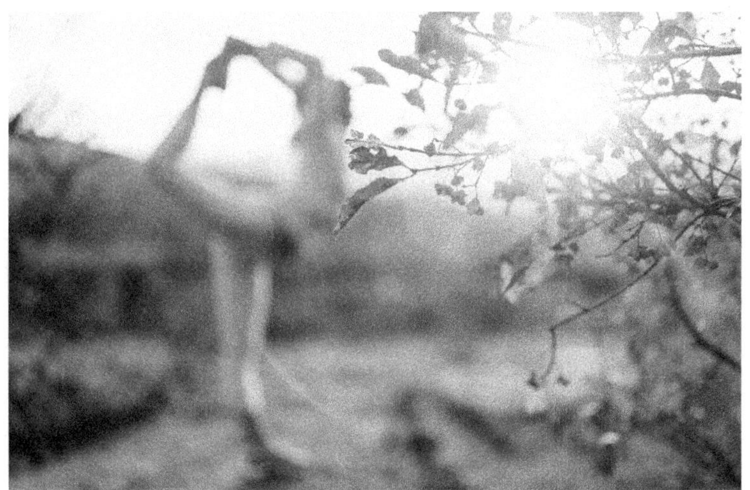

In addition to being vital for general well-being and self-assurance, maintaining proper posture is also very important for managing weight. Poor posture can affect energy expenditure, metabolism, and even food choices, which can lead to weight gain or impede efforts to lose weight. To effectively execute posture correction measures and support weight loss objectives, it is imperative to understand how posture influences weight management.

## The Impact of Posture on Weight Management

1. Metabolic Impact: The body's ability to efficiently use its metabolism is influenced by posture. Slouching or hunching over oneself can compress internal organs and hinder digestion, which slows down the metabolism and burns fewer calories. This may make it harder to keep off extra weight or maintain a healthy weight.

2. Muscle Engagement: The back, obliques, and abdominal muscles must all be actively engaged in order to maintain good posture. These muscles may weaken or become unbalanced when posture is poor, which lowers muscle tone and lowers caloric expenditure. Increasing calorie burning and supporting weight loss efforts can be achieved by strengthening these muscles with posture correction exercises.

3. Energy Expenditure: When engaging in physical exercise, proper posture encourages efficient movement and energy expenditure. Poor posture can cause inefficient movement, which raises the energy required for daily activities and exercise. People can support weight loss objectives by improving movement efficiency, conserving energy, and increasing calorie burning during physical exercise by adjusting their posture.

4. Appetite Regulation: An individual's posture might affect their appetite and dietary preferences. According to research, maintaining proper posture whether sitting or standing may have a positive effect on hormone regulation, particularly

those that regulate metabolism and hunger. People who keep an upright posture may find it easier to control their hunger, experience fewer cravings for harmful foods, and adhere to a nutritious diet, all of which are critical for managing their weight.

5. Emotional Well-Being: Mood and emotional well-being are greatly influenced by posture, and mood and emotional well-being can influence weight control activities. Feelings of exhaustion, worry, and low self-worth are linked to poor posture, and these factors can contribute to emotional eating, a decline in motivation for exercise, and trouble maintaining a healthy lifestyle. People can assist in long-term weight loss and improve their emotional well-being by adopting better posture and a positive body image.

**Including Techniques for Posture Correction:**

1. Awareness: Developing awareness is the first step toward good posture. Throughout the day, be mindful of your posture, particularly when sitting, standing, and walking. Take note of any routines or inclinations—such as rounding the shoulders or slouching—that lead to bad posture.

2. Posture Exercises: To strengthen your core muscles, realign your spine, and encourage better posture, include posture correction exercises into your everyday regimen. Planks, bridges, and shoulder retractions are a few exercises that can assist build stronger muscles and support proper posture.

3. Ergonomic Adjustments: To encourage good posture, make ergonomic changes to your daily routine and work environment. Make sure that your feet are flat on the floor, your chair provides sufficient lumbar support, and your computer monitor is positioned at eye level for an ergonomic workspace. Employ ergonomic add-ons like standing desks or lumbar cushions to encourage better posture all day.

4. Mindfulness Techniques: To develop body awareness and encourage relaxation, engage in mindfulness practices including deep breathing, meditation, and body scanning. Reduced tension and stress in the body can lead to better posture and more favorable weight management results. Mindfulness can help with this.

5. Professional Advice: For individualized suggestions and assistance with posture correction, think about consulting a physical therapist, chiropractor, or posture specialist. These experts are able to evaluate your alignment, spot any weak points or imbalances, and create a customized plan to meet your individual requirements.

Through comprehension of the relationship between posture and weight control and the application of focused posture correction techniques, people can bolster their attempts to reduce weight, improve general health, and elevate their standard of living. Prioritizing posture correction can have long-term advantages for mental, emotional, and physical health, which will ultimately lead to a happier and healthier way of life.

# Physical Activities to Enhance Postural Alignment

Through the release of chronic muscular tension, the reeducation of the neuromuscular system, and the promotion of increased body awareness, somatic exercises provide a gentle and comprehensive approach to improving postural alignment. You can treat underlying imbalances, reestablish natural movement patterns, and develop a more erect and aligned posture by implementing somatic techniques into your everyday routine. The following list of somatic exercises is intended to help with postural alignment:

**1. Shoulder Rolls: Somatic**
- Assume a comfortable stance, keeping your arms at your sides and your feet hip-width apart.
- Take a breath and raise your shoulders to your ears, tensing your upper trapezius muscles.
- Release your breath and roll your shoulders back and down so that your shoulder blades move easily along your rib cage.
- With each roll, concentrate on releasing tension from the neck and shoulders so that the muscles can extend and relax.
- Continue doing this exercise in multiple rounds, paying attention to your movements and letting your breath direct them.

**2. Spinal waves somatic:**
- Place your feet hip-width apart and bend your knees just a little bit.
- For support, rest your hands on your hips or the small of your back.
- Take a breath raise your chest and push your pelvis forward while arching your spine.
- Tuck your chin into your chest and tilt your pelvis back as you release the breath as you round your spine.
- Keep doing this flowing movement, gracefully transitioning with each breath from a backbend to a forward fold.
Pay attention to how the movement is flowing; let your spine move in all directions and let go of any tension with each wave.

**3. Physical Pelvic Stunts:**
- Lay flat on your back with your feet flat on the ground and your knees bent.
- To feel the movement, put your hands on your pelvis.
- Take a preparatory breath, then release it as you flatten your lower back into the floor by tilting your pelvis towards your navel.
- Take a breath to bring your body back to neutral and restore your lower back's natural arch.
- Carry out multiple repetitions of this exercise, syncing it with your breathing.
- Pay attention to releasing pelvic and lower back tightness so that the pelvis can move easily and organically.

**4. Chest Opener Somatic:**

- Maintain a lofty stance, keeping your arms at your sides and your feet hip-width apart.
- Straighten your arms and interlace your fingers behind your back to elevate them away from your body.
Breathe in as you feel a stretch across the front of your shoulders and chest as you open your chest and raise your gaze to the ceiling.
- Let go of the stretch and return your arms to your sides by exhaling.
Perform multiple rounds of this exercise, emphasizing chest opening and enhancing thoracic extension.

## 5. Hinge on the Soma:

- Place your feet hip-width apart and bend your knees just a little bit.
- For support, rest your hands on your hips or the small of your back.
- Take a breath and bend at the hips, bringing your chest forward and your tailbone back.
- Release your breath as you stand back up, using your core and glutes to help with the action.
- Carry out this hip hinge movement again, paying attention to keep your spine neutral the entire time.

## 6. Somatic Whole-Body Sensitivity Assessment:

- Extend your legs and keep your arms at your sides while lying on your back.
- To center yourself, close your eyes and inhale deeply several times.
- Start by focusing your attention on various body parts, working your way up to your head from your feet.

- As you scan every area of your body, take note of any areas that are tense, uncomfortable, or unbalanced.
- Let go of any tension with each breath and give your body permission to soften and relax.
- Keep doing this full-body awareness scan for a few minutes, giving yourself permission to inhabit your body completely and developing a sense of alignment and ease.

Try incorporating these somatic exercises into your everyday routine to help with tension release, postural alignment, and body awareness. You may help your body find its natural state of alignment and balance by mindfully performing these moderate motions. This will enhance your posture and general well-being.

# CHAPTER 8

## SOMATIC AWARENESS AND MINDFUL EATING

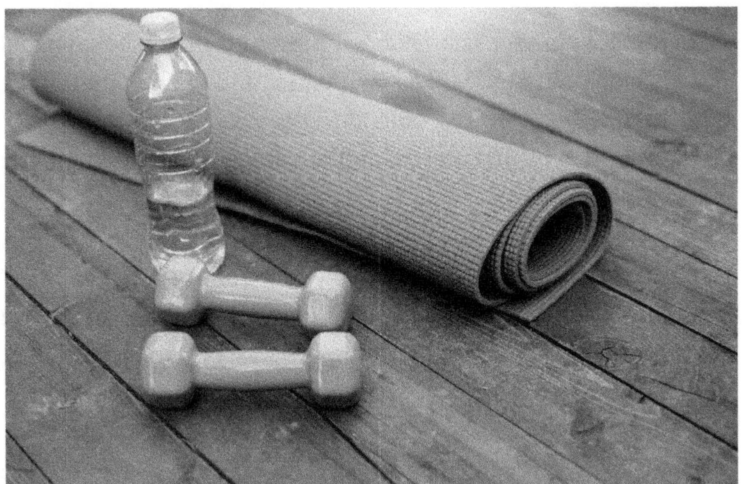

**B**y increasing awareness of hunger and satiety cues, encouraging healthier eating choices, and decreasing overeating, integrating mindfulness into eating habits can have a significant positive effect on our relationship with food. Mindful eating becomes even more potent when combined with somatic awareness practices, which center on tuning into bodily sensations and cues and allowing us to fully connect with the experience of eating and nourishing our bodies. Here's how to improve somatic awareness and develop mindful eating habits:

## Developing Insightfulness in Eating Behaviors

1. Involve Your Senses: Before biting into the dish, savor its flavor and aroma as well as its texture and even sound. Take note of the hues, forms, and designs present on your dish. Breathe in deeply the aroma, and relish the moment when you get to taste each bite.

2. Eat Distraction-Free: Reduce the amount of time you spend watching television, using your phone, or reading while you eat. Give your whole focus to the process of eating, allowing yourself to savor every bite's aromas, textures, and sensations.

3. Chew Slowly and Thoroughly: Savor the flavor and texture of the food by taking your time to chew every bite completely. Take note of your chewing and swallowing sensations, as well as the feel of the food as it passes through your throat and mouth.

4. Pay Attention to Your Body: Throughout the meal, pay attention to your body's signals of hunger and fullness. Keep track of when you start to feel satisfied and when you start to feel hungry. Eating should be done thoughtfully and slowly;

instead of eating more out of habit or peer pressure, stop eating when you are comfortably satisfied.

5. Gratitude Practice: Develop thankfulness for the food on your plate and the sustenance it gives your body. Consider the source of the food, the work involved in cultivating or preparing it, and the wealth of nutrients it provides to promote your overall health and well-being.

**Improving Somatic Sensitivity:**

1. Body Scan Meditation: Spend a few minutes closing your eyes and doing a quick body scan meditation before starting your meal. Start with your feet and work your way up to your head, bringing your awareness to every area of your body. In the current moment, allow yourself to fully enter your body by noticing any regions of tension, discomfort, or sensation.

2. Tune Into Hunger and Fullness: Become aware of your body's physical experiences of hunger and fullness. Take note of how food feels in your stomach before, during, and after eating. Rather than waiting until you are extremely hungry or eating past the point of fullness, try eating when you are moderately hungry and ending when you feel pleasantly filled.

3. Notice Emotional Triggers: Be aware of any emotional triggers, such as tension, boredom, or sadness, that may affect your eating habits. Take note of how these feelings show up as tension or other bodily sensations in your body. Prior to eating, release emotional tension and build a sense of peace

and presence by engaging in somatic awareness practices like progressive muscle relaxation or deep breathing.

4. Notice desires Without Judgment: Rather than resisting or passing judgment when desires emerge, notice them with compassion and curiosity. Examine other options to satisfy your needs without using food as a comfort or diversion, and pay attention to the feelings and ideas that go along with the craving. Recognize that it's acceptable to have cravings and that you have the ability to respond to them thoughtfully by practicing self-compassion and kindness.

5. After Eating, Consider Your Food Choices: After you've finished your meal, consider your food choices and the physical, mental, and emotional effects they had on you. Examine your eating habits for any patterns or tendencies, and think about how you may make more deliberate decisions that support your goals and beliefs for your health and well-being.

You can improve your relationship with food, strengthen your bond with your body, and create a more harmonious and balanced life by integrating somatic awareness techniques with mindful eating habits. You can develop a more attentive and satisfying connection with food that promotes your general health and well-being by viewing eating as a chance to nurture and take care of yourself.

# Improving Eating Awareness Through Somatic Practices

In order to improve our awareness of eating, somatic activities can help us become more attuned to our bodies, identify signals of hunger and satiety, and cultivate a more mindful connection with food. We can build better eating habits, strengthen our connection to the body's intrinsic knowledge, and enhance our general well-being by integrating somatic practices into our eating routines. Here's how to improve eating awareness with somatic practices:

1. Scan Your Body Before Eating:
- Spend a moment meditating on your body scan before a meal or snack. Shut your eyes and focus on every body part, beginning at your toes and working your way up to your head.
- Observe your body's tense spots, sore spots, and sensations. Observe your body's sensation in the here and now, without passing judgment or doing an analysis.
- You can start to develop a stronger awareness of your physical state and potential indicators for hunger or fullness by paying attention to your body's signals before eating.

2. Position for Mindful Eating:
- Be mindful of your eating position. Maintain a straight spine and relaxed shoulders when sitting comfortably. With your hands resting on your lap or the table, place your feet flat on the floor.
Take a few moments to perform a somatic check-in in order to decompress. Breathe deeply for a few moments, letting your

body unwind and come into a state of awareness and presence.

- You may foster a conducive environment for paying attention to your body's cues and enjoying the act of eating by taking up a mindful eating posture.

3. Involve Every Sense:

- When eating, use somatic awareness to stimulate all of your senses. Take note of the food's flavors, textures, and colors while it sits on your plate. Before you bite into your dish, pause to enjoy its aesthetic appeal.

- As you start eating, observe how each bite tastes, feels in your mouth and is heated. Chew carefully and gently, allowing your palate to slowly reveal the flavors and sensations.

- You can develop a stronger bond with the food you eat and improve the sensory experience of eating by using all of your senses.

4. Recognize your hunger and fullness cues:

- Use somatic approaches to become aware of your body's signals of hunger and fullness. Take a moment to check in with your stomach and note any physical feelings of emptiness or hunger before you eat.

- Observe how your hunger fluctuates when you eat. When you start to feel full or satisfied, pay attention to it and think about slowing down or halting to give your body time to register these feelings.

- You can learn to eat more intuitively and steer clear of overeating or undereating depending on outside cues by paying attention to your body's signals of hunger and fullness.

5. Conscientious Biting and Reflux:
- Develop an awareness of the chewing and digestive process through somatic techniques. Take note of your chewing and swallowing sensations, as well as the feel of the food as it passes down your throat and into your mouth.
- For the best possible digestion, chew every bite carefully and slowly, letting the flavors develop and the food crumbles into smaller pieces.
Increased nutrient absorption from the food you eat can be achieved by supporting your body's natural digestive process and raising awareness of the chewing and digestion processes.

6. Examine your body feedback:
- After eating, pause to consider how your body is feeling. Take note of any shifts in your mood, energy level, or bodily experiences.
- Think about how the food fed your body and if it gave you the desired energy and satisfaction.
You may learn a lot about how certain foods and eating habits impact your general well-being and make better decisions in the future by paying attention to your body's input.

Including somatic activities in your diet can improve your awareness of what you eat, encourage you to choose healthier foods, and help you develop a stronger relationship with your body's natural knowledge. It is possible to have a more attentive and satisfying relationship with food that benefits your general health and well-being by paying attention to your body's feelings, recognizing signs of hunger and satiety, and using all of your senses when eating.

# CHAPTER 9

# INCLUDING SOMATIC EXERCISES IN YOUR DAILY ROUTINE

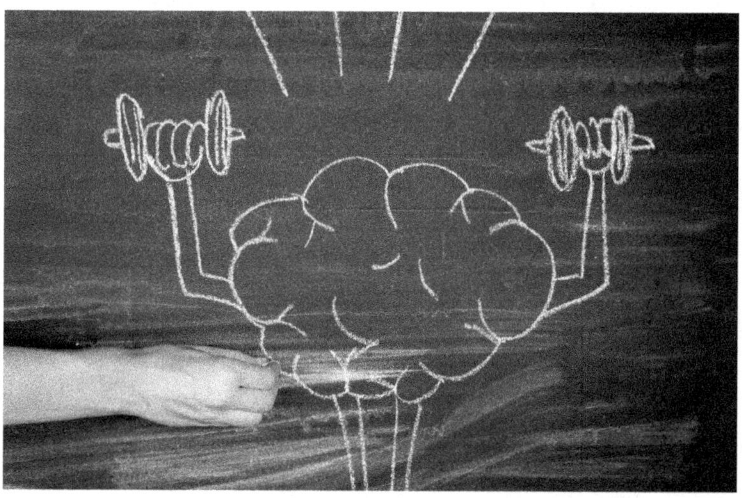

Including somatic exercises in your daily routine can have a significant positive impact on your general health by increasing body awareness, lowering stress in your muscles, and improving your range of motion and flexibility. You can benefit from these mild yet effective activities by designing a somatic workout regimen that works well with your everyday schedule. Here's how to include a somatic workout regimen into your everyday schedule:

1. Clarify Your Intentions:

- To start, make it clear why you want to include somatic exercises in your daily regimen. Establish clear objectives, such as stress reduction, posture correction, or increased mobility, and think about the ways in which somatic practices can help achieve these goals.

2. Begin Little:

- As you gain comfort and proficiency, progressively increase the duration and intensity of your somatic workout regimen. Begin with a sensible period of time. As your body adjusts to the techniques, start with shorter sessions each day and work your way up to longer ones.

3. Select Your Workouts:

- Choose from a range of somatic exercises tailored to your individual requirements and objectives. Incorporate activities aimed at relieving stress, strengthening body awareness, increasing mobility, and encouraging relaxation. Try out a variety of methods, including mindful body scans, breathwork, and slow movement sequences, to see which suits you the best.

4. Ensure Uniformity:

- Maintaining consistency is essential to benefiting from somatic workouts. Whether you want to do your somatic workout program before bed, during your lunch break, or first thing in the morning, set up consistent times throughout the day to do so. Maintaining consistency will support the routines and habits you're attempting to create.

5. Throughout the Day, Integrate:
Seek ways to incorporate somatic exercises into your regular routine. During the day, incorporate easy stretches and motions when you're waiting in line, sitting at your desk, and taking breaks. You may keep your attention on body awareness and relaxation throughout the day by incorporating somatic techniques into your regular routine.

6. Pay Attention to Your Body:
- Pay attention to the signals from your body and modify your somatic workout regimen as necessary. When performing a specific exercise, adjust the action or attempt an alternative approach if you feel uncomfortable or encounter resistance. Recognize the limits of your body and refrain from exerting more effort than you are capable of.

7. Engage in Mindfulness Practice:
- Be alert and present when performing your somatic workout regimen. Pay close attention to the feelings and experiences associated with every breath, movement, and instant. Develop an inquiring and accepting mindset regarding your body, enabling you to investigate and gain fresh perspectives with every exercise.

8. Track Development:
- Monitor your development and take note of any adjustments or enhancements to your physical, mental, and general state of health. Observe changes in attitude, posture, and flexibility as well as any

easing of stress or muscle tightness. Appreciate your accomplishments and make use of them as inspiration to keep up your somatic workout regimen.

9. Be Adaptable:
- Be adaptive and flexible when it comes to your somatic exercise regimen. There may be days when you're unable to finish your routine in its entirety because life can be unpredictable. Rather than giving up, come up with inventive methods to fit somatic practices into your day, even if it means cutting sessions short or altering your schedule to suit your needs at the moment.

10. Make self-care a priority:
- Prioritize your well-being by setting aside time each day to do somatic activities that will nourish your body, mind, and soul. Instead of seeing your somatic workout regimen as just another task to cross off your to-do list, see it as a chance to take care of yourself and refuel your energy. Making self-care a priority will support you in the long-term maintenance of a fulfilling and sustainable somatic practice habit.

You too may get the transformational benefits of these gentle yet potent practices by following these guidelines and incorporating somatic exercises into your everyday routine. Whether your goals are to live a more balanced and satisfying life, reduce stress, increase body awareness, or improve mobility, a regular somatic exercise program can promote your general well-being.

## Guides for Success and Maintenance Over the Long Term

With somatic exercises, long-term success demands dedication, regularity, and a conscious approach to self-care. The following advice will assist you in continuing your somatic practice and gaining long-term benefits:

1. Set Achievable Goals: Consider your present fitness level, way of life, and personal preferences when setting realistic goals for your somatic practice. Divide more ambitious objectives into more doable benchmarks, and acknowledge your advancements as you go.

2. Make Consistency a Priority: Long-term somatic exercise success depends on consistency. Establish a consistent timetable for your somatic practice and honor your commitments to make it an indispensable part of your weekly or daily schedule.

3. Listen to Your Body: During your somatic practice, pay attention to your body's input and modify your technique as necessary. Recognize the limitations of your body, refrain from overexerting yourself, and adjust any exercises or methods that are painful or taxing.

4. Remain Present and Mindful: As you engage in your somatic practice, pay close attention to the feelings, emotions, and experiences at every instant. Approach your practice with

curiosity and nonjudgment, allowing yourself to explore and gain knowledge from each session.

5. Practice Self-Care: Give yourself the attention and time you need to engage in physical, mental, and spiritual activities. Incorporate other self-care techniques like yoga, meditation, or enjoyable and relaxing hobbies in addition to somatic exercises.

6. Be Persistent and Patient: Acknowledge that it could take some time and patience to make improvements with somatic exercises. Practice consistently, even on the days when you don't feel motivated or up to par. Remain dedicated to your objectives and have faith in the process.

7. Seek Accountability and Support: Assemble a network of people who are understanding and supportive of your somatic practice journey. For more accountability and support, think about enrolling in a somatic exercise class or online group.

8. Mix It Up: Try experimenting with various exercises, methods, and adaptations to keep your somatic practice interesting and pleasurable. To keep your practice interesting and dynamic, mix up your stretches, motions, and breathwork.

9. Monitor Your Progress: Maintain a journal or log of your somatic practice sessions to monitor your development over time. Keep track of any adjustments or enhancements you experience in your posture, flexibility, mobility, or general well-being, and acknowledge your progress as you go.

10. Be Flexible:  Recognize that life can be unpredictable and be flexible and adaptable with your somatic practice schedule. If your schedule is off, come up with inventive methods to fit somatic activities into your day, even if it means cutting sessions short or changing your method.

You can achieve long-lasting improvements to your physical, mental, and emotional well-being by heeding these suggestions and being dedicated to your somatic practice. Keep in mind that somatic exercises are a journey rather than a goal and that every minute you spend in body connection offers you the chance to develop, heal, and transform.

# CONCLUSION

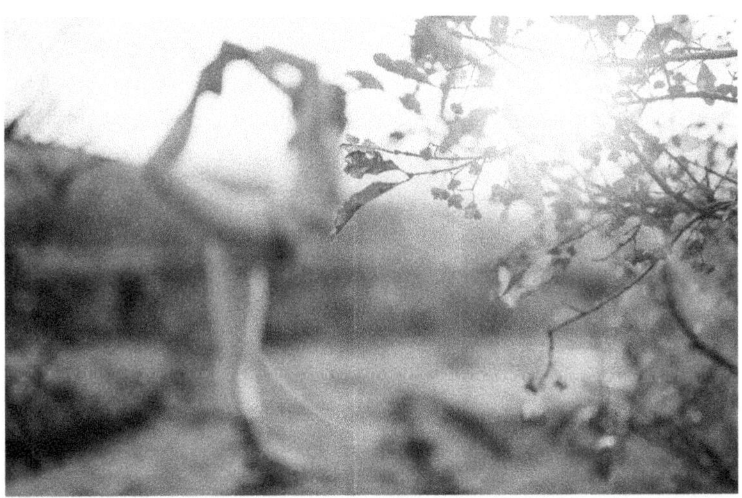

In summary, by encouraging increased body awareness, relieving tension, and promoting relaxation, somatic exercises provide a comprehensive strategy for improving physical, mental, and emotional well-being. We have covered a number of important ideas and techniques on this journey that will enable you to integrate somatic exercises into your regular routine and reap their life-changing effects.

## Key Concepts Recap:

1. Understanding Somatic Exercises: We now know that the main goals of somatic exercises are to retrain the neuromuscular system, encourage conscious movement, and

develop a heightened awareness of the sensations and motions of the body.

2. Advantages of Somatic Movement: There are several advantages to somatic exercises, such as better posture, increased body-mind connection, flexibility, mobility, and less stress.

3. Mind-Body Connection: Researching the relationship between our ideas, feelings, and physical experiences has shown how these interconnections affect our general health and well-being.

4. Somatic Exercise Principles: Our somatic practice has been led by fundamental ideas like mindfulness, breath awareness, and gentle movement, which have helped us develop a closer relationship with our bodies and the present moment.

5. Integration into Daily Life: Consistency, mindfulness, and self-care are key components of the practical tactics we've discussed for incorporating somatic exercises into everyday activities.

6. Long-Term Success: Lastly, we covered strategies for long-term maintenance and success, such as prioritizing self-care, setting reasonable objectives, remaining consistent, and paying attention to your body.

Remember that every somatic exercise practice session is a chance for personal growth, healing, and self-discovery as you continue on your journey. You can achieve significant transformation and improved well-being in all facets of your life by practicing mindfulness, listening to your body's knowledge, and remaining dedicated to it.

Accept the path, have faith in the procedure, and follow your body's intuition to live a life full of energy, harmony, and inner serenity.

## Encouragement for Continued Somatic Practice for Weight Loss

Starting a weight reduction somatic practice journey is a tremendous commitment to your health and energy. It's critical that you maintain your inspiration and motivation as you proceed, fostering your commitment to your somatic practice. Here are some words of motivation to assist you keep up the good work and accomplish your weight loss objectives with somatic exercises:

1. Appreciate Progress, Not Perfection: Keep in mind that each step you take to reach your weight loss objectives is an accomplishment and of celebration. Recognize and celebrate your accomplishments, no matter how tiny, and realize that every somatic practice session moves you one step closer to your final objective.

2. Embrace the Journey: See the development of your somatic practice as a continuous process of self-awareness and maturation. Accept the highs and lows, the victories and failures, as priceless chances for growth and change. Recognize that every hour you spend in connection with your body is a step toward better health and well-being, so have faith in the process and remain dedicated to your practice.

3. Listen to Your Body: Your body is a wealth of knowledge and insight that may help you achieve the highest levels of vitality and health. During your somatic practice sessions, pay attention to the indications and cues they give you, and treat their demands and limitations with kindness and

consideration. When it comes to your weight loss journey, pay attention to the subliminal cues of hunger, fullness, tension, and relaxation.

4. Build Self-Compassion: As you overcome the difficulties and roadblocks associated with weight loss, treat yourself with kindness and compassion. Since self-compassion is necessary for long-term adjustment and development, treat yourself with the same compassion and understanding that you would give to a close friend. Honor your body as a holy vessel deserving of care and nurturing by treating it with love and respect.

5. Rediscover Joy in Movement: Somatic activities present a special chance to rediscover the delight and joy of movement. Examine various somatic approaches, movement styles, and mindfulness exercises to find what makes you feel the happiest and most fulfilled. Discover activities that connect with your body and spirit, whether it's expressive dance, mindful walking, or gentle stretching, to bring joy and energy to your practice.

6. See Your Success: Take a moment to picture yourself reaching your weight loss objectives and leading a vibrant, vital life. Imagine yourself feeling light, strong, and invigorated in your body as you move with elegance, ease, and confidence. Utilize the power of imagery to encourage you to stay focused on your journey and to reaffirm your dedication to your somatic practice.

7. Remain Connected: Assemble a strong support system of people who share your dedication to somatic practice and weight loss objectives. Look for local gatherings, social media groups, or online forums where you may make connections with others, exchange stories, and lend support and encouragement. Having a community of supporters can provide you with the inspiration, accountability, and drive to continue practicing what you love.

Keep in mind that there is no one-size-fits-all strategy for weight loss and that your somatic practice path is specific to you. Have faith in the wisdom of your somatic practice, in your body, and in yourself to lead you to a better state of health, happiness, and well-being. You have the ability to reach your weight loss objectives and build the vibrant, satisfying life you deserve with commitment, tenacity, and a strong connection to your body. Continue to shine brightly while you go somatically!

# Scan QR Code to Access Free Bonuses and Join Our 30 Day Challenge.

## HOW TO SCAN QR CODE

To scan a QR code, take the following general actions:

**1. Open the Camera App**: The majority of contemporary smartphones come with a built-in QR code scanning feature in their camera apps. Open the camera app on your smartphone.

**2. Set the Camera Position**: Slightly shake your phone and aim the camera toward the QR code you wish to scan. Verify that the well-lit QR code is inside the frame.

**3. Scan the QR Code**: The QR code ought to be instantly recognized by your smartphone's camera app. It could provide a link or a notification to access the content linked to the QR code.

4. **Follow the Prompt**: After the QR code is detected, adhere to any on-screen instructions. This could include clicking on a link to visit a website, downloading an application, or seeing particular content.

**5. Access the Content**: You ought to be able to view the content linked to the QR code after scanning it and following any instructions. This might be a website, an electronic voucher, contact details, or other kinds of information.

You might need to enable the QR code recognition option in your smartphone's settings or download a QR code scanning app from the app store if the camera app on your phone isn't picking up codes automatically. You should consult your device's user manual for more details since certain devices might have unique motions or instructions for reading QR codes.

# A 14-DAY WORKOUT PLAN

**14-Day Somatic Exercise Plan for Weight Loss**

**Somatic exercises** focus on mindful movement and body awareness, promoting overall well-being and potentially aiding in weight loss. This plan incorporates a variety of low-impact somatic exercises suitable for different fitness levels.

## Plan Structure:

- **Frequency:** The plan suggests daily workouts, but adjust based on your needs and listen to your body. Rest is crucial for recovery and progress.
- **Duration:** Each workout is approximately 30 minutes.
- **Warm-up and Cool-down:** Each session commences with a 5-minute light cardio warm-up (e.g., walking, gentle jumping jacks) and concludes with a 5-minute cool-down (e.g., gentle stretches, breathing exercises).

*Day-by-Day Breakdown:*

**Days 1-3:** Focus on **foundational movements and body awareness**

- **Pelvic tilts:** Lie on your back, knees bent, and feet flat. Gently tilt your pelvis up and down, engaging your core muscles. Repeat 10 times in each direction.
- **Cat-Cow:** Start on all fours, hands under shoulders, and knees under hips. Inhale, arching your back and looking up (cow pose). Exhale, rounding your spine and tucking your chin (cat pose). Repeat 10 times.
- **Arm circles:** Stand with feet shoulder-width apart. Make slow, large circles with your arms, forward and backward, for 10 repetitions each direction.
- **Leg swings:** Standing or holding onto a chair for support, gently swing one leg forward and backward, maintaining a small range of motion. Repeat 10 times each leg.

**Days 4-6:** Introduce **gentle strengthening exercises**

- **Squats:** Stand with feet shoulder-width apart and toes slightly outward. Slowly lower yourself as if sitting in a chair, keeping your back straight and core engaged. Stand back up with control. Repeat 10 times.
- **Lunges:** Step forward with one leg, lowering your body until both knees are bent at 90-degree angles. Push back up to the starting position, alternating legs. Repeat 10 times per leg.
- **Plank:** Start on your forearms with elbows under shoulders. Keep your body in a straight line from head to heels, engaging your core. Hold for 30 seconds, gradually increasing duration as you get stronger.

- **Side Plank:** Lie on your side, propped up on one forearm. Lift your hips off the ground, forming a straight line from head to feet. Hold for 30 seconds per side.

**Days 7-9:** Focus on **balance and coordination**

- **Single leg stand:** Stand on one leg, holding onto a chair for support if needed. Maintain good posture and hold for 30 seconds, alternating legs.
- **Heel-toe walk:** Walk heel-to-toe for 30 seconds, focusing on maintaining balance and controlled movement.
- **March in place:** High knees march for 30 seconds, followed by 30 seconds of butt kicks, maintaining good form.

**Days 10-12: Increase intensity and incorporate variations**

- **Repeat exercises from previous days, increasing repetitions or hold times slightly.**
- **Incorporate additional exercises like arm raises, leg lifts, or gentle twists, focusing on controlled movement and deep breaths.**

**Days 13-14: Active recovery and reflection**

- **Go for a light walk or do gentle yoga.**
- **Focus on deep breathing exercises and meditation.**
- **Reflect on your progress and how you feel. Adjust the plan as needed for the following week.**

**Additional Tips:**

- **Stay hydrated by drinking plenty of water throughout the day.**
- **Eat a healthy, balanced diet to support your weight loss goals.**
- **Listen to your body and take rest days when needed.**
- **Consult a certified fitness professional for personalized guidance and modifications if needed.**

Remember, consistency is key! Stick to the plan, listen to your body, and enjoy the journey towards a healthier and more mindful you.

www.ingramcontent.com/pod-product-compliance
Lightning Source LLC
Chambersburg PA
CBHW070818280726
48660CB00016B/2119